Fit Moms for Life

How to Have Endless Energy to Outplay Your Kids

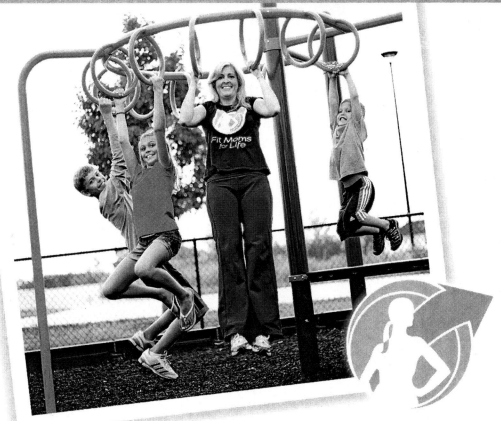

DUSTIN MAHER

Fit Moms for Life

How to Have Endless Energy to Outplay Your Kids

By Dustin Maher

Note to reader: Consult with your physician before beginning this or any exercise or nutrition program.

ISBN 978-1-61448-080-8 Paperback
ISBN 978-1-61448-081-5 eBook
Library of Congress Control Number: 2011933170

Published by:
MORGAN JAMES PUBLISHING
5 Penn Plaza, 23rd Floor
New York City, New York 10001
(212) 655-5470 Office
(516) 908-4496 Fax
www.MorganJamesPublishing.com

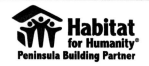

In an effort to support local communities, raise awareness and funds, Morgan James Publishing donates one percent of all book sales for the life of each book to Habitat for Humanity.
Get involved today, visit
www.helphabitatforhumanity.org.

Acknowledgements

There are so many people I want to thank and acknowledge. Without their work, this book would have never gone from my mind to paper. In order not to show any favoritism, the following acknowledgments are in no particular order.

I want to first start by thanking YOU. Yes, you. Thank you so much for investing the time to read this book. It means so much to me that you would take the most valuable resource we have on earth—time— and spend it with me.

Next, I would like to thank the thousands of clients I have been blessed to train and work with over the past years. If it weren't for your willing spirits and your consent to be my "guinea pigs," I wouldn't have been able to determine the best workouts, eating plans, and motivational strategies to get maximum results. Thank you for your sweat, determination, and never-quit attitudes. You inspire me, and I can't thank you enough.

In particular, I want to thank the 30+ amazing women you will meet in these pages: You represent what this book is all about—unwavering commitment to your goals, an unwillingness to settle for second best, and an ability to put all five pillars of health and fitness together. Without your stories, this would be just another "how to" book, but thanks to your incredible transformations, it takes on a whole new meaning and will most definitely inspire countless others, showing them that success isn't just possible, but only a matter of following the plan.

I want to go way back to my high school days and my 11th-grade English teacher, Mrs. Sandusky. Thank you for encouraging me to write, even though I hated to do it and was awful at it. Your kind words and encouragement meant a lot and helped me to not give up writing altogether.

Next, I want to thank my family for their support: my dad, for telling me that anything is possible and to chase after my dreams; and my mom, for showing me selfless love throughout the 19 years I was at home, and for always being there. Thanks to my three siblings, Chris, Angela, and Eric, for sibling rivalry and support growing up. Thank you to my girlfriend, Abby, who has put up with my drive to finish this book and let me make it my main focus.

This book was in my heart for a couple years before the actual finished product appeared. If it weren't for Cailin O'Connor, it may never have been completed. Thank you, Cailin, for all your hard work on this project, for seeing my vision, for keeping the book in my voice, and for helping me choose my words in a coherent way so that they can change lives. I would also like to acknowledge five editors who took a look at the book and helped me tighten some sections and expand others: Thank you, Vanessa Beardsley, Tiffany Chapin, Anne Daugherty-Leiter, Lisa Janis, and Becky Nelson. Thank you to my copy editor Josh Wimmer and graphic designer Katy Smith.

Thanks to Tracie Hittman Fountain for helping so many of my clients throughout the years heal their metabolism and look and feel their best. Thanks for contributing your eating plan to this book.

Thanks to Luke Severson and Althea Dotzour for taking the wonderful pictures you see in the book, to Jody Rindy for her willingness to model for the exercise photos, and to Kim Richter and her kids for modeling for the cover photo.

Shifting gears a little bit, I would like to thank Mary Kay, a company that I have looked up to for many years. I am so impressed by your ability to empower women and help them see their own potential. The community that you have built is a great example that I hope to be able to replicate with the *Fit Moms for Life* communities. In particular, thanks to Lisa Madsen of Mary Kay for being an example of a great leader who keeps her life balanced yet is constantly going after her goals.

Thanks to the amazing blogger Janice Croze, for seeing my vision and sharing that vision with her large following at *5minutesformom.com.*

A big shout out to Holly Rigsby of Fit Yummy Mummy for helping me when I was just starting out and being an awesome example of how to create an amazing group of women and how to build a powerful community. I am very impressed and grateful for the guidance.

I am very thankful to have a great publisher in Morgan James Publishing. Thank you to Rick Frishman for all your support and the motivation to write this book. Thank you to Steve Harrison for teaching me how to use this platform I have been given to share my message of hope with others.

Thank you, Ryan Lee, for mentoring me and encouraging me to not just think of myself as a trainer, but as an information and ideas person—someone who can change lives with his words. Also a big shout out to Jim Labadie, Pat Rigsby, and Nick Berry for their help in growing my fitness business and for creating one of the best supplement companies around in Prograde.

Thank you to my more recent coaches, Bedros Keuilian, Craig Ballantyne, Steve Hochman, and Chris McCombs, for believing in me, encouraging me, challenging me, and keeping me accountable. But most of all, for teaching me to dream big.

Thank you to Tim Ferriss, one of the most brilliant thinkers of all time, for helping me promote this book and get it into as many hands as possible. I hope to someday repay you for all the help you have given me.

I know Tony Robbins gets tons of shout outs, but Tony, thanks so much for dedicating your life to empowering and coaching others. Although I have not yet met you, your words, written and spoken, have taught me that obstacles are only bumps in the road toward success. I have gone through your programs countless times and will continue to do so. Keep up the great work.

Similarly, I would like to thank Steve Linder for taking me under your wing, helping me out with my business, and giving me a greater understanding of how the mind really works and how our thoughts affect our behaviors.

On the topic of coaches, a big thanks to Brendon Bruchard for taking time to invest in my life and for encouraging me to tell my story. I am so drawn to your passion and your ability to be "present" at all times. I hope we meet again soon.

Last and certainly not least, I would like to thank my Lord and Savior Jesus Christ for blessing me with certain talents and abilities and helping me see, from a relatively young age, what my mission in life entailed. I am certainly not perfect and struggle every day, but Your grace and Word help me through.

Table of Contents

Chapter 1: Becoming a Fit Mom for Life   **1**
Fit Moms for Life Transformations:
    Jody   9
    Becky   10
    Jennifer   11
    Kelly   12

SECTION 1
MINDSET: COMMITTING TO BE FIT FOR LIFE

Chapter 2: Change Your Mind, Change Your Body   **15**
Fit Moms for Life Transformations:
    Trish   23
    Marsue   24
    Vanessa   25
    Tina   26

Chapter 3: Goal Setting   **27**
Fit Moms for Life Transformations:
    Abby   31
    Sandra   32
    Elizabeth   33
    Laura   34

Chapter 4: Getting Real   **35**
Fit Moms for Life Transformations:
    Karen B.   48
    Liz   49
    Jenny   50
    Patty   51

SECTION 2
NUTRITION: EATING TO BE FIT FOR LIFE

Chapter 5: Food as Fuel   **55**
Fit Moms for Life Transformations:
    Amber   78
    Jane   79

Chapter 6: Making It Work   **81**
Fit Moms for Life Transformations:
    Crystal   90
    Katy   91

SECTION 3
STRENGTH AND BURST TRAINING: MOVING TO BE FIT FOR LIFE

Chapter 7: Lifting in Order to Tone   **95**
Fit Moms for Life Transformations:
    Sarah   107
    Donna   108

Chapter 8: The New Rules of Cardio   **109**
Fit Moms for Life Transformations:
    Karen E.   114
    Lynn   115

Chapter 9: Putting Together an Exercise Routine   **117**
Fit Moms for Life Transformations:
    Lynda   134
    Mary   135

SECTION 4
ENVIRONMENT: STAYING FIT FOR LIFE

Chapter 10: Fit Mom, Fit Family   **139**
Fit Moms for Life Transformations:
    Alecia   146
    Patrice   147

Chapter 11: Creating Your Fitness Community   **149**
Fit Moms for Life Transformations:
    Aimee   157
Fit Moms for Life Communities:
    North Dakota   158

Chapter 12: Your Transformation   **159**
Fit Moms for Life Transformations:
    Nancy   161
    Tiffany   162

APPENDICES

A: Fitness for New Moms and Moms-to-Be   **165**
B: Documenting Your Journey   **171**
C: Resources for More Information   **179**
D: Frequently Asked Questions   **181**
E: Dustin's Workout DVD Programs   **189**

About the Author   **193**
Free Bonus   **195**

Becoming a
Fit Mom for Life

Kristin is arranging the carry-ons in the overhead compartment with a crying 2-year-old on her hip as she assures her 5-year-old that Bunny doesn't need a seat belt on the plane. She pulls out a coloring book for her 7-year-old and a sippy cup for the toddler just before it's time to get everyone buckled in for takeoff. Kristin and her kids are on their way to meet her husband in Florida to visit his parents. Her husband has been away at business meetings for the past three days. She's hoping her in-laws might watch the kids one night, so that she and her husband can go out for a nice dinner.

Traveling is definitely stressful with three kids. Life in general has become so overwhelming that it's hard to think beyond getting through the day.

"I am so burnt out," Kristin thinks. "I feel like I just give, give, give."

Her husband travels a lot and works long hours when he is home, so she is basically taking care of the kids alone most of the time. Every day she gets everyone up, dressed, and fed, and performs taxi duties to school, sports, and other extracurricular activities. Some days she takes the youngest to the babysitter so she can work at the part-time job she started recently, after her husband's pay was cut. Other days she takes care of her toddler, runs errands, does the grocery shopping, and stops in to visit her parents. They're getting older and have some health issues, and she's the only one living close enough to take care of them. Evenings are busy, with dinner to fix and dishes to do, homework to help with, baths, and then story time and kisses. Folding the laundry while she watches her favorite show is as close as she gets to "me" time anymore. Packing for this trip was a stark reminder that she still hasn't lost the weight from her last pregnancy. All those cute warm-weather clothes that used to fit are still boxed up, waiting for the weight to miraculously fall off.

Kristin feels the tears well up as the flight attendants begin their safety speech. She's heard it a hundred times before, but for some reason today is different. Maybe it's because she's so exhausted or because it just hit home how crazy her schedule is. Maybe it's because her kids are all sitting quietly doing their own thing, for once.

For whatever reason, it hits her hard: "In the rare event that the plane loses cabin pressure, oxygen masks will fall down from the ceiling. To start the flow of oxygen, pull the mask toward you. Place it firmly over your nose and mouth, secure the elastic band behind your head, and breathe normally. Make sure you have safely secured your mask before assisting those around you."

Kristin freezes. "That's it!" she thinks. "That's my problem. I go through life helping everyone else, but forgetting my own oxygen mask!" Her lack of patience with the kids, her distance from her husband, and her exhaustion all stem from having come last on her own list of priorities for far too long. "Things are going to change," Kristin thinks. "They have to, starting now."

I wrote this book for you and all the moms, like Kristin, who feel like they've lost control of their lives. I know you never feel like you have enough time, energy, confidence, or passion. I know it is draining to be the caregiver to everyone in your life: your kids, your husband, your boss, your parents, your friends, your church, and your neighbors. I hope you are beginning to realize that you've done so much and helped so many people, but that you aren't helping yourself.

Here is my question for you: If you don't help yourself, who will?

"But, Dustin," you're saying, "you don't know my life. I don't have time to work on me. Look at all these people who count on me and the situations I have to deal with!"

> *What started out as something for my own health really has impacted my whole family. We all eat better now. My daughter is learning about health. My energy level and happiness level have really increased. I'm able to handle stress better. I don't yell as much. So you can think of it as something you're doing for yourself and for other people."*
>
> – Elizabeth

You're right; I don't know your situation. But having worked with thousands of women, I can guarantee that all areas of your life will improve when you put yourself first and start taking care of yourself.

Your relationship with your kids will be better because you'll have more energy to play with them and more patience when they misbehave. You will be a better wife or partner because you'll have more confidence and less stress. You will be a better contributor at work because you'll be able to think more clearly. You will be a better volunteer at church or in your community because you'll have greater self-awareness and more confidence in your abilities.

Are these big promises?

You bet.

I invite you to take this wild journey with me, and I will deliver on these promises. This journey requires you to say, "I deserve the best for me." This is not about being selfish. It's about being your best so you can be at your best for others.

Are you ready? Let's go!

Fit Moms for Life

This book is designed to help you get into the best shape of your life and get endless energy. You're not going to do it just by eating well and exercising the way I describe—though that's a big part of it. You're going to transform your body and your life by learning to take care of yourself, finding your motivation, setting meaningful and challenging goals, and surrounding yourself with other people who help you achieve those goals.

A lot of my clients have told me this is what sets my program apart from all the other fitness and weight-loss programs out there: the focus on the entire person. I interviewed 31 of my clients who have undergone amazing transformations. You'll see a couple of their success stories at the end of each chapter and hear from them throughout the book. (Look these women up on my website to see more of their stories.) You'll see that in addition to their amazing physical improvements, these women have become more confident and more comfortable with themselves. They've set goals for themselves that go way beyond weight loss and fitness. They are pursuing and reaching their goals today and setting new ones for tomorrow.

> *I think what makes Dustin's program unique is that there really is a focus on the life goal. It's not just about dropping pounds or taking off inches or getting stronger. It's really about taking control of your whole life and using exercise as a piece of that."*
>
> *– Lynn*

Whether you're a new mom who's trying to figure out how to still be "you" now that your days are filled with diaper changes and lullabies, or an experienced mom wondering what life will hold now that your kids are getting older, this book is for you. If you're currently pregnant, hope to get pregnant soon, or recently had a baby, this book is for you, too. Appendix A, "Fitness for New Moms and Moms-to-Be," will help you stay healthy throughout pregnancy and get back into shape after your baby is born. And while this book is written for moms, my sound exercise and nutritional advice is just as useful for women who don't have children—and for men. Anyone can use this program to get into the best shape of their lives.

My Background

My interest in fitness started when I was growing up in Minnesota. I was a decent athlete in high school, but not a great one, and I was pretty scrawny. But I loved sports, and I really enjoyed eating healthy. My mom was very smart when it came to nutrition. She was always teaching me and my three siblings about nutrition, helping us make healthy choices and being a good role model for us.

I left home to attend the University of Wisconsin–Madison. I had decided in first grade that I was going to be a weatherman, so I started out majoring in meteorology. Meanwhile, my love for fitness continued to grow. Living away from home for the first time, I was eating healthy food because I wanted to, not because my mom was cooking it for me. I was also learning more and more about exercise, and I found I enjoyed teaching others about it when I visited home.

When I went back for my sophomore year, I switched my major to kinesiology, or exercise science. I started working at the rec center on campus, enrolled in the personal training program there, and became certified as a personal trainer. During this time I started teaching fitness classes, which was a lot of fun. After a while, I got the opportunity to work at a health club. I graduated in 2006 and have been working full time as a fitness professional and building my own fitness business ever

> *Dustin's program is the best investment you will ever make in yourself and your life. It is a real program based on science and based on the information that he knows that will help you to get the best body for you."*
>
> – Crystal

since. I developed MamaTone classes and another program called Fit Fun Boot Camps, which has grown into one of the largest boot camp programs in America. Between group class participants and clients in one-on-one and small group training, I've worked with more than 5,000 people and helped them to lose tens of thousands of pounds and reach their fitness goals. Since releasing my first fitness video in 2008, I've sold more than 10,000 DVDs to clients around the world.

Why I Work With Moms

A lot of people find my career choice surprising. I'm a young guy, with no kids of my own, and yet I'm passionate about helping moms achieve optimal fitness. I think there are a few different reasons for it.

First, I'm very close with my mom. My parents are still together after 32 years. I'm the oldest of four kids and my mom was a stay-at-home mom. Her days were filled with meeting our needs and maintaining the house. I always thought she was awesome. She gave, gave, and gave of herself—and she never put herself first. I didn't think about it as a kid, but looking back as an adult, I can see she didn't give herself the time she needed. I see so many moms who are overworked and often underappreciated, whether they're staying home with their kids or working outside of the home.

Another reason I work with moms is that I just enjoy it! While I was in college, I got a lot of satisfaction out of training professors and university staff who were moms. I also trained some of my mom's friends, mostly postmenopausal women, and I really enjoyed that, too. Most of the moms I've trained bring a lot of energy to their workouts, and they really appreciate having that time to focus on themselves and their health. When they get results, they're so proud of themselves, and their kids are proud of them, too.

> " The program is so well researched. It works and it's clear that it works. It's not a fad thing—the results that people have gotten are long-term. I feel like Dustin is thinking about the whole person and what people will need. And it's real."
>
> – Tina

I also love the fact that I'm influencing the next generation by working with moms. I've only been doing this for six years, so it's too early to tell, but I anticipate that kids who are raised by active, healthy, confident moms will be a lot healthier and confident in their own lives. So by helping the mom, I'm helping her kids...and maybe even her husband, though that can be a tougher sell!

My Fitness Philosophy

Different fitness professionals have very different perspectives on what people should do to achieve their optimal fitness. I'm not saying my way is the only way. There are many ways to get in shape and to stay in shape, but what I can tell you is that my program works. **It's an approach to fitness that is well rounded and sustainable, and one busy moms can fit into their lives.** It is not a gimmick or a fad or a magic pill that promises results without effort.

My program is built around five pillars of health: **mindset, nutrition, strength training, burst training, and environment.** You might be able to get some results in the short term by just focusing on one or two of these areas, but you'll get your greatest results, and make them last, when you incorporate all five. I'm going to cover each of these pillars in detail throughout this book, but for now let's just look at the big picture of what each one means.

- **Mindset.** Mindset is the most important aspect for someone who wants to change her life and her fitness level. You've got to believe that you can make a change and that you're worth it. So many people have negative attitudes toward healthy eating or exercise. They feel like they're going to be overweight no matter what they do—so they don't do anything. And so many people, especially moms, don't believe that they're worth it. They put everyone else's needs above their own and neglect their own health. With that kind of a mindset, it will be really tough for you to get in shape and keep in shape. In Chapters 2, 3, and 4, I'll help you get into the right mindset, identify the negative beliefs that are holding you back, set realistic and motivating goals, and assess your starting point.

- **Nutrition.** You've got to eat healthy. People think they can eat poorly if they work out enough—but as most people find out the hard way, that just isn't true. I've seen so many people try this, but they all learn that their body is not going to change that much through exercise alone. I want you to eat a good combination of whole foods, in small portions, 4-6 times a day. In Chapters 5 and 6, I'll share some basic rules about eating and nutrition, meal and snack ideas, and recipes, as well as tips for how to stick with a healthy diet.

- **Strength training.** I'm a big fan of strength training using heavy weights and I've seen it help hundreds of women get into the best shape of their lives. Contrary to popular belief, running marathons or doing long-distance cardio doesn't help your body burn fat and keep it off. In fact, I believe that traditional cardio makes you fat. Obviously, you have to build up to lifting heavy weights and do it safely, but my program is about pushing yourself to your max—which means leaving those five-pound dumbbells behind. In Chapter 7, we'll go through the exercises you should be doing to build muscle, burn more calories, and tone your entire body, so that you'll be excited to bare your arms when summer comes along. I'm even sharing the exact exercises from the first DVD in my *Fit Moms for Life* series in Chapter 9, so that you can start exercising and seeing results right away.

Five Pillars of Fitness—in My Clients' Words

Mindset: *"I used to mentally talk myself out of doing things. And now I totally believe in myself in ways that I never ever had before. I have faith, and I know I am capable of anything I want. I'm living a healthy, happy lifestyle and taking care of myself because I'm worth it."* – Abby

Nutrition: *"I've never looked at food the way I see it now. I see it as fuel for my body. I have really found that food is the secret behind becoming the best athlete I can be and the best, happiest person I can be."* – Liz

Strength training: *"Don't be afraid to lift heavy weights. You will be surprised at how much you can lift if you work up to it, and with good form. And you won't bulk up."* – Donna

Burst training: *"With burst cardio, it is over with quickly and you burn those calories really fast. You don't have to go out and run for an hour. It's so beneficial for the shape of your body and your strength."* – Karen E.

Environment: *"I really notice that the choice of people who I spend time with is different. They are people who support me in my goals. And I support them in theirs. There are other people who might want the old Aimee back, so we can go out to lunch and order the cheese fries—and I don't see them as much anymore. When people say they want to spend time with me, I'm like, 'Well, come work out with me.'"* – Aimee

- **Burst training.** As I already said, I don't recommend traditional cardio, which raises your heart rate moderately for long periods of time. (This is referred to as "steady-state cardio" in the fitness world.) Burst training is much more effective and efficient. With burst training, you exercise at a very high intensity for a short duration—anywhere from 10 seconds up to maybe a minute—and then you rest or go to a lower intensity to bring your heart rate back down. Then you bring it back up for that short duration again, and go back and forth for five, 10, 15, maybe 20 minutes. (You may have heard of "interval training" before. That's a similar philosophy, but it uses more gradual transitions. Burst training is more intense and more effective.) I'll tell you more about burst training in Chapter 8 and describe different ways to include it in your exercise routine in Chapter 9.

- **Environment.** The final piece of the puzzle is environment. This is really key to maintaining the changes you make in your mindset, nutrition, and exercise routines. The good news is that, as a mom, you have a lot of influence on the environment within your home and your family. More likely than not, you make most of the decisions about what foods come into your house and what activities your family engages in. You can switch your weekly "movie and popcorn night" to "dance party in the living room night," and you can choose to spend snow days with your kids sledding instead of baking (and eating) cookies. But you also need to look at who you're spending time with, how you spend your free time, and how you entertain yourself. You have to make an effort to be part of a fit family and a fit community – in Chapters 10 and 11, I'll tell you more about how to do that.

My Mission and Vision

My mission—and the reason I'm writing this book—is to reach one million moms by the end of 2015 with the support they need to change their mindset, eat better, exercise effectively, and be part of fit families and communities so they can transform their bodies and their lives. My vision is a nationwide network of fitness programs that will function like support groups for moms. Each group might be set up a little differently.

> *You feel like you're in it together. You want to motivate each other. You want to push each other, but you want to celebrate your successes together, too, which I really enjoy."*
>
> – Jennifer

Some will be large groups, others will be very small. Some will meet several times a week to work out together, with occasional meetings to discuss nutrition or just to socialize and support each other. Others will work out on their own and come together less frequently to share information and support, and communicate online between their meetings to keep each other accountable. I call these groups *Fit Moms for Life* communities. I'll go into more detail about what a *FMFL* community looks like in Chapter 11.

The reason I've chosen this mission is that I've seen how much power deep, authentic relationships have when it comes to helping people to transform their lives. I feel those relationships are what is missing—not just in our current approach to fitness, but also in our society as a whole. I believe that by sweating together, pushing each other to succeed, and holding each other accountable, moms can develop unique bonds of a type many people don't experience in today's world. By providing a structure for moms to get together, really get to know each other, and build relationships that last, I hope to ignite a movement of moms who are passionate about putting themselves first, transforming their bodies and lives, and empowering other women to do the same.

I also believe that the most important things we can do in life are to empower others, share our knowledge, and motivate others to reach their goals. Each of us is limited in how many people we can reach. But if I can reach you, and you can reach five of your friends and family members, and they can each reach another five, that million-mom goal won't be so far off. Please check my website at *fitmomsforlife.com* to learn more about *FMFL* communities worldwide and to learn how you can get involved.

On the next pages, you'll find four of my clients' transformation stories. These stories are placed at the end of each chapter to help you see what is possible when you take the information in this book and apply it to your life. My goal is for these stories to motivate, educate, and inspire you.

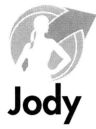

Fit Moms for Life Transformation

Jody

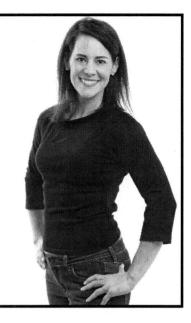

Jody's had amazing results from my program and is in the best shape of her life, despite giving birth to five kids! She is a great example of how a busy mom can make it work, and is featured in DVD 1 of the *Fit Moms for Life* series.

Jody's story: "I was never a really fit person, just kind of short and stocky. After giving birth to my fifth child at 34, it was really difficult to lose the baby weight. I'd lost the weight after my other kids by just watching what I ate and running a little bit. But this time around it was really, really hard, and I was frustrated. Running wasn't working, my diet wasn't working, and I wasn't seeing what I wanted to see. I started going to Dustin's MamaTone classes when my youngest was six months old. My husband said it would be better to spend the money on the class than on buying more clothes in a bigger size!

"The first week I hurt very badly; I'm not going to lie. But I kind of thought, 'If it hurts this much, it's got to be doing something.' So I came back and started seeing a difference more quickly than I had in anything I'd ever done before.

Jody, 37, mother of five, including twins. 5'3", 117 pounds. She has lost 70 pounds through my program.

"That was three years ago. I can do 50 push-ups and eight pull-ups. It's like I'm a totally different person. People look at me like, 'Jody's fit? Jody's in shape? What the...?' It's nice when my husband puts his arms around me and can wrap around more than once. He is also very appreciative. Let me just clarify that right now: He's liking it."

Jody's nutrition tips: "There are so many websites for healthy dinner ideas. I know a lot of moms struggle to come up with a healthy dinner every day for their families, but it's easy to just search for 'healthy dinners' and find something. It's not hard. You just have to discipline yourself to do it."

Jody's advice to you: "Try it. I mean, really, what are you going to do just sitting there? Nothing. Just try it. Give it six weeks. I don't know anyone who's done Dustin's program for six weeks and hasn't seen results."

Read more of Jody's story at *fitmomsforlife.com/jody*, and work out with her in Chapter 9 and on the first *Fit Moms for Life* DVD.

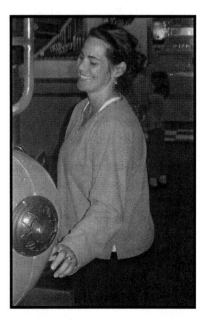

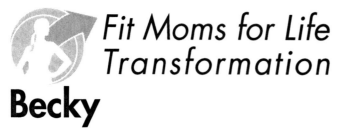

Fit Moms for Life Transformation

Becky

Becky's story is very much about overcoming obstacles and doing what you can with what you've got. Despite numerous health challenges, she has radically transformed her body and her life.

Becky's story: "I won't go into my whole medical history, but I have lupus, arthritis, endometriosis, hypothyroidism, celiac disease, and migraines. I also have a chronically ill son, and I had postpartum depression after he was born. So I had plenty of excuses when I started putting on weight and not getting rid of pregnancy weight. It took me awhile to admit it, get serious, and do something about it.

"Since my medical issues really limit the use of my legs, most traditional exercise programs don't work for me. I can't really do any cardio because of problems with my knees. But with Dustin's program, I can keep my heart rate in the aerobic range through strength training. When I first started, I could barely do a push-up against a wall. Now I do push-ups with my hands on a stability ball and one foot on a chair.

"It is amazing what the weight training has done for me. My body is totally transformed. Despite my ongoing medical problems, I have more energy to be active and do things with my kids now."

Becky's exercise tips: "You have to work through whatever else is going on. I work through my fatigue when I haven't slept because I've been up with my son. I'll feel a migraine coming on, and I work through it. You'd think it would send me in the wrong direction, but it gets the endorphins going, and it almost always gives me more energy and helps me feel better. I've actually had migraines that didn't get full-blown because I exercised when I felt them coming on."

Becky's advice to you: "Do it now. Don't wait. Don't say you'll do it next week or when you finish your deadline. I always thought my life was going to change, and that I would get in shape once things got easier. But you never know what is actually going to happen, and the only time to start is now."

Read more of Becky's story and see a video of one of her in-home workouts at *fitmomsforlife.com/becky.* And see her in the upper-body workout portion of *Fit Moms for Life* DVD 11.

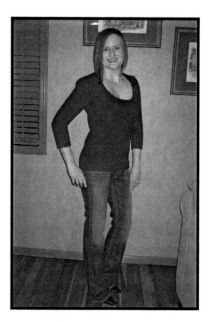

Becky, 39, mother of two. 5'5", 123 pounds. Becky overcame significant physical challenges to lose more than 50 pounds, drop from a size 18 to a size 4, and cut her body-fat percentage in half— all by lifting heavy weights and doing no cardio at all.

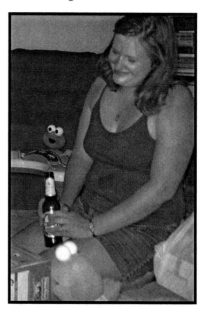

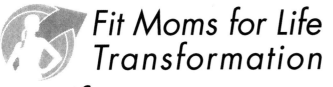

Fit Moms for Life Transformation

Jennifer

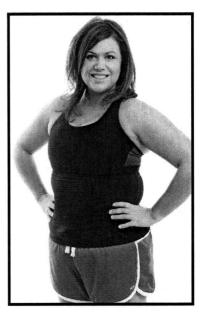

Jennifer is one of my first clients to hit the 100-pound weight-loss mark, and she continues to work incredibly hard. She is really goal-oriented and competitive, and I love that she is always setting new goals for herself.

Jennifer's story: "A year ago I was at my highest weight ever. I don't know exactly what I weighed, because I was embarrassed to even step on the scale, but the one time I did weigh myself, it said 278. I would guess I was 285 or more when I decided that this was not the way I wanted to live. I was staring down turning 30. I didn't work out. I didn't think much about what I ate. I was an emotional eater. And just a very different person than I am today.

Jennifer, 30.
5'8", 182 pounds.
Jennifer lost 100 pounds and went from a size 20/22 to a size 12 in about a year following my program.

"Comparing my life to how it was a year ago, it's like night and day. When I started boot camp, I couldn't even do a push-up on my knees. Everything felt like a struggle. I would get winded going upstairs. Now I can do 40 real push-ups. This past weekend I easily went on a five-mile run with my boyfriend. I could not have fathomed that a year ago. I'm also just a lot happier. I have a more positive outlook. I used to carry a lot of shame, not just about how I looked but about who I am. I'm in a serious relationship now, and I think that has to do with my confidence in who I am as a person."

Jennifer's current goals: "My long-term goal is to weigh 140. I have a short-term goal for running sprints on the treadmill. Right now I'm doing 25 seconds on, 35 off, at 15 percent incline and a speed of 7.5. I'd like to get to 30-30 doing that, and increase my pace to eight miles per hour. I also want to do a triathlon this summer."

Jennifer's advice to you: "Don't let fear hold you back. Think about what you want to change, and then set a goal for tomorrow or for today. It can be something little. Not everything has to happen in one day. You just have to start taking a first step."

Read more of Jennifer's story at *fitmomsforlife.com/jennifer.*

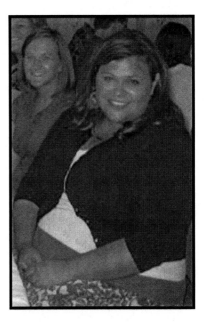

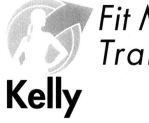

Fit Moms for Life Transformation

Kelly

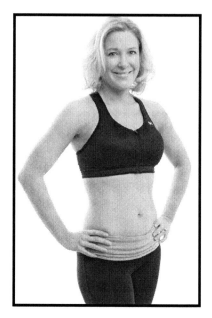

Kelly is one of the more fit moms I've worked with. She got her college body back after having two children. She's one of the few people who can actually do Level 8 of my *Got Core* DVD!

Kelly's story: "After having two babies in less than two years, I would try to fit exercise in, but I thought there just wasn't any time to do it. By the end of the day I was so exhausted that I couldn't bring myself to pop in a video. I was fed up with the way I felt and the way I looked. I had a picture in my head of how I looked back in college, and I was tired of not being that person anymore.

"The thought of getting up at five in the morning for boot camp was daunting. I didn't think I would be able to work out that early and get through the day. But I've found that working out early gives me more energy for the rest of the day.

Kelly, 33, mother of two. 5'4", 123 pounds. Kelly lost more than 25 pounds and three dress sizes doing my boot camps.

"I also have a lot more confidence. Sometimes I can't believe that I'm now a size 4, because I was a size 8 or 10 for as long as I can remember. When I walk into a room, I no longer feel like people are staring at me thinking, 'Wow, she has really let herself go.'" Instead, I get noticed for being fit! This added confidence has helped me in my career as an attorney.

"I was diagnosed with hypothyroidism after the birth of my first child. Hypothyroidism is a condition that slows your metabolism and was an added weight-loss challenge. Even now, I have to work out extra hard and have to be very careful with my eating to maintain my weight."

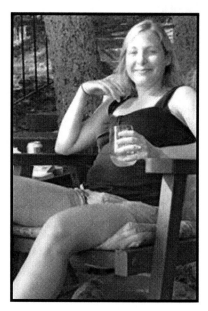

Kelly's advice to you: "No one else can really push you or tell you that you need to do it. You just need to decide for yourself that this is the time you are going to make a change. And it will work."

Read more of Kelly's story at *fitmomsforlife.com/kelly*, and work out with her on the *Buns, Guns, Back & Shoulders* DVDs.

MINDSET: COMMITTING TO BE FIT FOR LIFE

"A lot of it is that inner drive, you know? You have to really want it to do it. Starting is really hard, but just be consistent—and once you start to see results, it gets easier." – Katy

"I think the first step is just knowing that you're worth it and stepping out the front door and doing something for yourself." – Liz

"I had to come to the realization that I was worth the boot camp price tag. That wasn't easy to do, since I was a stay-at-home mom and I wasn't contributing financially to our already modest household income at the time. I needed to believe that I was worth the time and the financial stress, and thankfully, my husband agreed with me." – Vanessa

If you're a mom, you've probably watched a child learn how to walk—or you will soon. Think of all the effort that an infant puts into learning how to crawl, to stand on his or her own, to walk with support, and finally, to take those amazing first independent steps. It takes so much focus and concentration to build up to that point. But within a month or two, the toddler is walking around, even running, without giving it a second thought!

That's how it is, to some degree, with getting your life turned around and getting healthy. It takes a lot of energy and hard work at the beginning as you try to change your habits. You have to dig deep to find the motivation to start, and it takes real dedication to pull yourself up to a standing position, find your balance, and feel confident enough to put one foot in front of the other, figuratively speaking. But once you start to see the results of all those efforts, it gets a little bit easier. As your new, healthy behaviors turn into habits, it takes less and less of your focus. If you're restructuring your environment to support those new habits, you're like that toddler—cruising around and barely even thinking about it. But breaking those old habits can be very challenging at the beginning, so we're going to take some time to get you started.

Before we get into the nutrition and exercise details of my program, it's important to put in some time reflecting and planning. The next three chapters are designed to help you figure out where you're going, why you're going there, and where you're starting from. Getting started is the hardest part, and I want to help you get started from a solid foundation that will make it easier to stick with the program over time.

Chapter 2 is all about changing your mindset so that you can change your body and your life. Get ready to spend some time reflecting and recording those thoughts. (You'll find pages to document your journey in Appendix B.) In Chapter 3, you'll have a chance to write out your goals after I describe what useful goals look like and why they are so important. In Chapter 4, I'll walk you through how to make a realistic assessment of your current fitness. It's impossible to know whether you're making progress if you don't know where you started!

If you're itching to get going with the program, you can skip ahead to the eating plan and the exercise routine and get started today! But I urge you to come back and read this section—soon—so that you can be sure you're starting in a way that will set you up for success. You'll notice I'll never tell you that my program is the only one that works. It's probably not a good thing to say from a marketing perspective, but the truth is that a lot of programs can be effective if you commit to doing them and then keep it up. What's truly unique about this program is that it is designed to fit into a busy mom's life, and it helps you address the things that get in the way of sustaining healthy changes in your life. So take the time to reflect on your mindset, your goals, and your starting point—because it's not just about what you eat and what kind of exercise you do. It's about how you find and maintain the momentum you need to become a *Fit Mom for Life*.

Change Your Mind, Change Your Body

Why Mindset Matters

I've spent a lot of time studying how results come about and why some people don't get the results they want. So much of it depends on beliefs and attitudes. Your thoughts create your actions. So you really have to change the way you think if you want to make significant changes in your life.

When it comes to fitness and weight loss in particular, a lot of people have negative attitudes about exercising, about eating well, about how possible it is to really change their bodies. People also hold very limiting beliefs about what they are capable of doing—both physically and mentally, when it comes to willpower and their ability to stick with a plan.

And like Kristin, the mom I talked about in the first chapter, a lot of women put their own needs on the back burner while they focus on taking care of everyone else. You have to believe that you're worth it and start putting yourself first to ensure that you're at your best—and that you'll continue to be able to help all those other people who depend on you.

If you're like most people and most moms, we need to start with your mindset before you'll be ready to commit to changing your life.

You Have to Really Want to Make a Change

When I meet a client for the first time, the first question I ask is: "Do you want to get in shape?" It seems like a strange question to ask someone who's just scheduled an appointment with a personal trainer or showed up for a boot camp, but I've found that a lot of people's answers aren't very convincing. Many of them just want the feeling of being in shape. They have this vision of themselves in better shape, maybe looking and feeling as good as their sister or their friend who's really fit. But that doesn't mean they're actually ready to put in the work and make the changes they have to in order to get in shape. And until they start to really want it, they aren't going to make the sacrifices they have to make and put in the hard work to get from point A to point B.

There's been substantial research on what has to happen before you decide to make a change in your life and stick with it. What it comes down to is that your current state has to be more painful for you than you imagine it will be to change. This can be about mental pain or about physical pain. Usually, it's a mix of the two.

Smoking is a great example of this. Smokers know that it will be painful to try to quit—going through withdrawal and losing that connection with the other smokers in their lives. They also know about the risks they're taking by smoking, but those risks seem sort of abstract and statistical if smoking isn't causing them any serious pain right now. Something has to happen to make their current state seem more painful than the perceived pain of quitting. Maybe it starts to get hard to breathe as they walk up a hill, or perhaps a friend or family member gets cancer. Maybe they're ready to start a family and they know about the negative impact smoking will have on their child and even on their ability to get pregnant. On the more extreme side, maybe it's a diagnosis of lung cancer or emphysema and a doctor telling them their life is on the line. In any case, suddenly something changes. The pain of quitting doesn't seem as bad as the pain they're currently in, or the pain they can now imagine themselves going through if they continue to smoke.

This scenario is the same for all kinds of changes people consider making—quitting a job, leaving a relationship, moving to a new city. And it's definitely the case for changing exercise and eating habits.

Once I know someone really does want to get in shape, my next step is to understand why they want to. I like to ask, "Why are you coming to see me now instead of six months ago or a year ago?" I want to understand their deeper motivation—not just "I want to lose weight" or "I want to feel better." Sometimes their deeper motivation is connected to what I talked about above—their current situation has become painful for them in some way. For a lot of moms, once we get down a little deeper, it's that they want their husbands to be proud of them and to love them and find them attractive. They want to be a good role model for their kids and to teach them healthy habits. They want to have the energy to keep up with their kids and to be around to enjoy their grandkids. They want to be a good example for their circle of friends or for a specific person in their life. Do any of these thoughts sound familiar to you? The emotions attached to those deeper, more personal motivations create the leverage to help you make changes and stick with them.

The 10-Year Plan: Create a Vision of Your Future

Knowing what it takes for people to commit to making a change, I like to do an exercise with new clients that I call the 10-Year Plan. This is a way of helping you envision where you want to go and where you don't want to go—and it can be very powerful in helping you stick with the changes you make.

Close your eyes and think about how your life will be 10 years from now if you continue with your current negative behavior. Obviously, we all engage in some healthy behaviors and some unhealthy ones. For now, let's just focus on the negative ones. If you continue living the way that you're living right now, how will your life look in 10 years? Take a few seconds to think about this. What would it look like? How would you feel? What would you be able to do—or what would you not be able to do that you can do now?

For example, maybe your lifestyle and the way you've been eating have caused you to gain weight pretty consistently over the last 10 years. Think about what another 10 years of weight gain will do to your body and your life. Maybe right now, hiking up a mountain is pretty tough for you. In another decade, going up two flights of stairs might be very difficult. Right now, you aren't fitting into your pre-baby clothes. In 10 years, you might not fit into an airplane seat, or be able to sit in the bleachers for your child's basketball game. Or maybe you have an 18-month-old and barely have the energy to keep up with him or her. If you don't change something, would you be able to have more kids like you've always wanted?

> " *Don't let the weight loss be your motivation, because once you reach that weight loss you will say, 'Oh, I lost my 40 pounds. I can go back to the way I was'—and that's how you regain the weight. But think about what you want to do with your life and what you minus 40 pounds will allow you to do— and let that be your motivation."*
> – Crystal

Get as graphic as you can. Put as much emotion into this as you can. Remember, we're trying to make this painful! Maybe there's a person in your life who has poor health or limited mobility because of lifestyle choices they've made. Think about whether you want to be like that in 10 years. When I talk with women in their forties or fifties, many of them say, "I don't want to be like my mom. She's in her sixties or seventies, and she can hardly do anything." On the flip side of that, picture how your kids will think of you as they get older. Are your kids going to look at you and think, "I never want to be like that"? Are your grandkids going to think of you as "old" and weak?

Now that you've visualized that, go to the 10-Year Plan exercise on page 172 and write it down. Write down how you'll feel, how you'll look, what you'll struggle with, and what your kids will think of you if you continue on your current path. You might even want to write more in a separate journal—spend 10, 15, 20 minutes journaling if you can, so that you really create a powerful image of what your life will be like if you don't take care of yourself.

Okay, that's the first part of the exercise. Now we're going to contrast that and think about a positive vision for the future, where you're living the healthiest life you can imagine. Snap your fingers and change the course your life is taking. If you start putting yourself first, taking care of yourself, and making healthier choices, what will your life look like in 10 years? Now that you've changed those negative behaviors and started taking care of yourself, what will you be able to do that you couldn't in your negative vision? Will you be able to hike that mountain that's a challenge today? How will you feel? Where will you be able to go? What will you be able to wear? Who will you get to see? How does that make you feel? What kind of joy will all these things bring to your life? What kind of mother, grandmother, friend, sister, or wife will you be? Think about it for a while, and attach emotion to it just like you did with the negative vision a few minutes ago. Meditate on it and think about how much more fulfilling your life will be when you make these changes.

After you've thought that through, go back to the 10-Year Plan exercise and write down the positives you visualized and the corresponding emotional images. Just like with the negative vision, the more detail you can imagine and write down, the better.

Now that you've done this exercise, you can see two distinctly different futures for yourself. I hope the first one was very negative and the second one was very positive, because that is what will motivate you to make a change and stay on a positive, healthy path. There will be times you don't want to get up in the morning to exercise. There will be times you just don't feel like planning your meals for the week. You have a cold, or you stayed up too late working on PTA business. You're traveling for a week and that gives you an excuse to eat less healthfully. But if you have these positive and negative visions of your future in mind—or even better, if you have them posted on your refrigerator so you see them every day—you can keep yourself motivated and get yourself back on track if you start to slide.

My client Trish started coming to boot camp after her sister was diagnosed with breast cancer. Her sister's illness made Trish realize the path she was on was not a healthy one. It was suddenly very easy for her to picture a future she knew she didn't want. She educated herself about cancer and nutrition and started exercising to take off her excess weight. "I knew I had to do this if I wanted to do anything in the future," she told me. That motivation is what keeps Trish going even now. "Any time I don't want to get out of bed or I don't want to go to boot camp, I think about my sister Bec," Trish said. "She always loved to run and get out and be active, but she can't do it anymore. So, it's like, I can get out and do it, and I have no reason not to. That keeps me going."

How to Get in the Right Mindset

Believe you're worth it. The first thing you need to do to change your mindset and get started on this path is to start to believe you're worth it. It's very basic, but you have to believe you should take the time for yourself. If you don't believe you deserve the investment in yourself, you're not going to put in all the effort this change is going to take. You're not going to get up early to exercise before the kids wake up, or pack your food at night to take to work the next day. You're not going to ask for the help you need from your husband or your family to make these changes. Our modern lives are so full of temptations, so full of opportunities to be lazy. If you aren't really committed, it's way too easy to fall off the wagon. Changing your life and your body is going to take hard work and consistency, and you have to believe you're worth it.

Put yourself first. Once you believe you're worth it, you need to learn to put yourself first. Not all the time, and not to the exclusion of taking care of other people—but you have to learn how to take the time you need for yourself and make sure you're getting your own needs met. A lot of moms seem to think that what they need is never as important as what everyone else needs from them.

I see so many moms who have ended up in a place where they don't feel good about themselves. They gain weight, they have low self-esteem, they start to feel cranky or have less patience with their kids, or they're more emotional. They thought they were being unselfish by putting everyone else in front of themselves, but in the long run, they weren't able to be as good a mom, wife, or friend as they wanted to be.

I'm not talking about ignoring everyone else around you or becoming an egomaniac. By putting yourself first, I mean you should be giving yourself 30 to 45 minutes a day, most days of the week, to take care of yourself. If you can give yourself that, you're going to find that

> " You'll be a better mom and a happier person if you just take a little bit of time for yourself."
> – Liz

you're less tired and more productive the rest of the day. Many people think they don't have the time to exercise—but once you put that time in, you're going to be able to think more clearly, and you'll be more efficient and effective in whatever else you need to do. Once you start seeing the benefits, your attitude will go from not having the time to not being able to afford to miss the workout.

Believe change is possible. The next thing you need to do to change your mindset is to believe change is possible. Most American adults have gone on diets. Unfortunately, studies show that after they stopped dieting, between one-third and two-thirds of them gained back even more than they had lost.[1] Many people have gone on an exercise kick at some point in their lives, but didn't see great results—probably because they either weren't eating correctly, or weren't building lean muscle, or both. If you've been through those situations or just witnessed others who have, you're probably skeptical about whether this program will work. That's why I'm including so many success stories in this book. I want you to see that this really does work—and that it has worked for someone like you.

You've got to tell yourself that if you put the time into it, if you follow the program, if you eat the right foods, if you change your environment, you will see results. You just have to start believing that when you put in the work, the results will come. Every once in a while, some doubt will sneak into your mind. Stay on track by rereading the *Fit Moms for Life* transformation stories that resonated the most with you and reminding yourself that you can do this—that change is possible.

---

1 Mann, T., et al. "Medicare's Search for Effective Obesity Treatments: Diets Are Not the Answer." American Psychologist 62.3 (2007): 220-33.

Practice positive thinking and speaking. Many people underestimate the power of positive thinking. Positive thinking leads to positive beliefs, positive actions, and positive results. I recommend that you develop and practice positive affirmations that will train your brain to think positively. It might seem a little hokey, but I've seen so many lives changed by it. I see a lot of moms who have very low self-esteem. They say they're ugly or that they don't deserve to be fit or that they've just let themselves go. They worry that their husbands don't find them attractive anymore and that they're being a bad influence on their children. Positive affirmations help them to overcome those negative thoughts and begin to see themselves in a more positive light. When you think and repeat these positive statements over and over again, they become part of who you are, and you're more likely to make decisions that are congruent with those beliefs.

I suggest you come up with five or 10 different positive affirmations that speak to you. They will be different depending on your situation and what kind of negative thoughts you are trying to overcome. One that I like to do or say is, "Every day in every way I'm getting stronger and stronger." "Stronger and stronger" can mean a lot of different things, whether it's mentally, physically, emotionally, spiritually, or something else meaningful to you. You might choose something as simple as "I am beautiful and worth it" or "Today is the day I make the healthy decisions to change my life." You can write your positive affirmations on page 173.

One technique is to write positive affirmations on index cards or Post-It notes and put them where you can see them—around the house, in your car, on your computer monitor. Pick a time at least once every day that you're going to read them aloud. You should also go over them in your head throughout the day. For example, you could post them around your house, and each time you see one, just take a couple of seconds to read it, either quietly or aloud. Saying it aloud may be even more effective.

> " I had a big fear that I just couldn't do the exercise. The voice in my head was really loud: 'You can't do it.' 'Who do you think you are?' 'There's no way you can do this.' And I had to just stamp that out."
> – Nancy

I also like to choose a positive statement to repeat while I'm exercising. During my burst training, or even sometimes when I'm lifting weights, I like to repeat a phrase that has a beat to it and kind of move to the beat. The more I do it, the more I say it, the more fired up and focused I get and the more I can push myself.

Many books have been written on positive thinking. This is just a brief overview. If you tend to have a lot of negative thoughts running through your head, I'd recommend you start reading or listening to books on positive thinking and speakers like Tony Robbins who talk about how to think positively.

Understand and overcome what's holding you back. Whether it's because of bad past experiences with diets and exercise or because they're dealing with trauma from their past, some individuals have something holding them back from achieving their potential and making the kind of transformation they could if they followed my program.

A lot of people have tried to lose weight before and failed. They may have negative associations with exercise or with eating healthy. Maybe you hated gym class as a kid and were always the last one picked for the kickball team. Maybe you've tried extreme diets before that were impossible to stick with. It's easy to get bogged down by those negative experiences and the negative beliefs that stem from them. Even though you may not have succeeded in the past, today is a new day and this program is something you can do. You're going to succeed this time if you do the right things. Take a few minutes to reflect on those negative beliefs, acknowledge them, and understand them—and then leave them behind.

Sometimes people are afraid of success. I see that frequently with people I've worked with and with people who comment on my blog. I've heard people who are overweight, and especially people who are morbidly obese, say that they're kind of hiding behind their fatness. They don't want the world to see who they really are. They've been hurt before, and they feel like if

> " As I began changing my lifestyle, I had to find different ways to connect with people I used to go out to eat with or engage in other unhealthy eating habits with."
> – Crystal

they lost that excess weight, they would be more vulnerable to being hurt again. If there's an issue like this holding you back or you feel like you're hiding behind your weight, you may need professional help to resolve those issues as part of your physical and mental transformation.

Get rid of negative influences and limiting beliefs. As you reflected on what is holding you back, you may have identified some negative influences in your life and some of your own negative, limiting beliefs. Once you've identified those, it's time to start getting rid of them—or at least reducing your exposure to them.

If there is a person or group of people in your life who are dragging you in the opposite direction of your goals, it might be appropriate to cut back on the amount of time you spend with them or how much you allow them to influence you. If your social life revolves around going out to eat and drinking excessive amounts of alcohol, try to schedule get-togethers of a different type. Work out with friends or go for a walk together, or go out for lunch at restaurants that offer some healthy choices. Bring healthy appetizers along when you go to watch a football game at a friend's house. Some of your friends might be grateful for a different way of socializing. Others will probably resist, and you won't see them as often.

It's more difficult when the negative influence is coming from your family members. I wouldn't suggest you cut off contact with your family, but you might need to make some changes in your relationships so that they don't have as great an influence on you. Let them know what you're working on and that you'd like their support. If they're not able to support your desire to get healthier, you might need to distance yourself from them somewhat.

The other thing we all need to work to overcome is our own limiting thoughts and beliefs. We've already talked about needing to believe that change is possible and overcoming negative experiences with exercise or healthy eating. But you probably have other limiting thoughts that you need to overcome. Just like positive thoughts lead to positive changes, negative thoughts will lead to negative actions and effects. Do you think of yourself as "big-boned" and believe you'll never truly change the shape of your body? Do you hate running (or some other particular form of exercise) and think you can't do it, even for a minute or two? Do you think you hate vegetables? When you read the transformation stories in this book, do you think that's great for those women, but that they're different from you somehow? They're not. So many of my clients held beliefs like these when I first met them, but they've overcome them and have seen fantastic results. So can you.

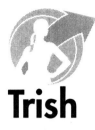

Fit Moms for Life Transformation

Trish

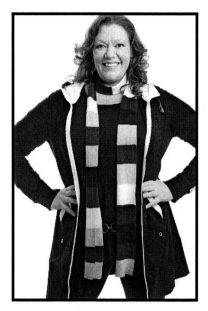

Trish decided to take her health into her own hands and became an avid exerciser. She's made an amazing internal and external transformation and has even started doing roller derby.

Trish's story: "I put on about 50 pounds over a couple of years after my second child was born. I stopped weighing myself when I was around 287. With boot camp and changes to my nutrition, I've taken off 70 pounds in the last two years. I went from a 24W to a regular 16. I'm out of the realm of 'women's sizes' and specialty stores.

"I used to do cardio at the gym, using the elliptical for 25 minutes a few times a week. I always referred to myself as the fittest fat chick, because I felt like I was fit but I was obviously very fat. The cardio I was doing was just not working. I felt powerless, because I didn't know what changes to make to my workout or my diet.

"My sister was diagnosed with cancer in December 2008. That was a really stressful time. I was in a downward spiral. I started to learn about the connection between cancer and nutrition. I changed how I was eating and lost almost 25 pounds. In May 2009, my friend Mo heard about boot camps and thought trying something different and exciting might be what we both needed. I'm absolutely hooked on it now. It's taken me to a whole new level in terms of what the second half of my life is going to involve. And I'm in it for life now."

Trish's nutrition tips: "There's a really short book that helped me a lot called *The Breast Cancer Prevention Diet* by Dr. Bob Arnot. People often feel like there's nothing women can do to prevent breast cancer, like it's just looming out there for us no matter what we do. But the premise of this book is that there are things you can eat to prevent breast cancer. Lo and behold, it turns out to be the same diet you should eat if you're diabetic, if you have heart trouble, or if you want to lose weight."

Read more of Trish's story at *fitmomsforlife.com/trish*.

Trish, 42, mother of two. 5'10", 217 pounds. Trish lost 70 pounds and increased her "good" cholesterol (HDL) count by 34 percent by doing boot camps.

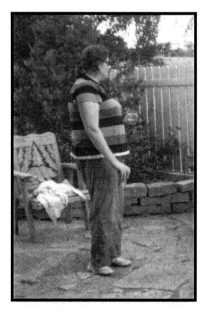

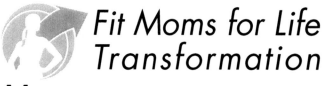

Fit Moms for Life Transformation

Marsue

Marsue's transformation is one of the coolest ones I've been a part of. She is virtually unrecognizable from her "before" picture and has gone on to become certified as a personal trainer!

Marsue's story: "I met Dustin when I went on one of his grocery store tours. I had already lost about 30 pounds at that point, but I was looking to do more. I started going to his boot camps, and it opened up a whole new chapter in my life. Once I achieved my weight goal, I decided the next step in my fitness journey was to help others achieve their goals. I got my ACE certification, I am now a trainer for Dustin's boot camps, and I have started a couple of my own fitness classes. I spend a lot of my free time looking up new exercises and trying new kinds of exercise.

"When I was heavier, my mindset was so different. I used to pass up going to weddings with my husband because I didn't want to be seen in public. I didn't want to have to put on a huge dress and look like a tent. I'm still an introvert, but I'm not down on myself anymore. It's like night and day."

Marsue's nutrition tips: "One: Get all the junk out of the house. If it's there, you're going to eat it. Two: Make sure you're getting all your water in. Three: It's not just about eating the right foods, but also portion control and spacing out your meals during the day. Four: Make sure you're eating your proteins and carbs together."

Marsue's exercise tips: "One: Don't be afraid to lift weights. You're not going to bulk up! You have to build that metabolism. Once you get that going, it's really going to help you. Two: Figure out what type of exercise you really like to do. And three: Mix it up, don't give up, and just have fun."

Marsue's advice to you: "Really look deep inside. Are you ready to make a change in your life? If you're ready to take that step, just do it. Don't be afraid."

Read more of Marsue's story at *fitmomsforlife.com/marsue,* and work out with her in *Fit Moms for Life* DVD 2.

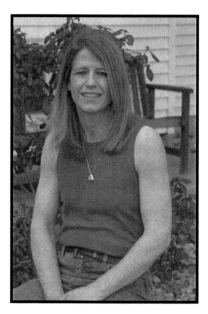

Marsue, 47, mother of one. 5'3", 120 pounds. Marsue went from a size 18 at 200 pounds to a size 4, and discovered her passion for fitness.

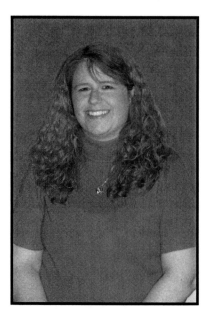

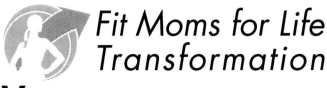

Fit Moms for Life Transformation

Vanessa

Vanessa is one of my boot campers who has made big changes not just physically but also emotionally. She's really focused and driven and willing to push herself.

Vanessa's story: "I took awhile to 'get to know' Dustin before starting his program. I got his newsletter for a year, and then I signed up for the *Fit Moms for Life* DVDs and worked out on my own for about five months. I finally joined boot camp in late 2009. Within the first three weeks I felt like a brand-new person. I had more energy, my outlook was more positive, and I had more patience with my kids. I felt more confident in a swimsuit and naked with my husband. When I started, I was 36 and my goal was to be the fittest I've ever been by 40. I reached that goal in less than a year. At 38, I am literally in the best physical, mental, and emotional shape of my life.

"Before Dustin's program, I had been clinically diagnosed and treated for depression and anxiety. I manage my depression and my anxiety with diet and exercise now. I no longer take any medication for those issues. I went off the meds almost immediately when I started boot camp. I just drew a line and decided this was how I was going to handle things. Around the same time, I discovered I have hypothyroidism and have since worked that out, which I think has made a huge difference, too.

"One of the less measurable things is that I can now show up at boot camp and push myself to my personal max and be okay with that effort. I don't get caught up worrying about how I compare to other people or what they think, and that's huge for me. I've never had a lot of self-confidence. I spent a lot of my life comparing myself to other people and always feeling like I came up short. And I don't feel that way anymore."

Vanessa's advice to you: "Dustin provides all the tools—a framework we can all tap into. The only variable in the equation is the person doing it. If you commit to doing your personal best, results will come. If you work, it works."

Read more of Vanessa's story at *fitmomsforlife.com/vanessa*.

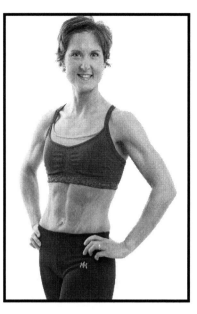

Vanessa, 38, mother of two. 5'3", 109 pounds. Vanessa lost 55 pounds and got on top of her depression and anxiety through my boot camps.

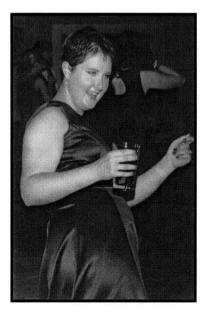

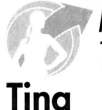

Fit Moms for Life Transformation

Tina

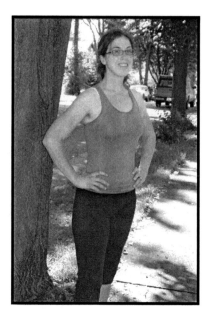

Tina is pretty new to my program, but I've been amazed at how quickly she shrank down and changed the shape of her body through my boot camp and fixing how she eats.

Tina's story: "It's always been a struggle for me to get exercise into my life. I'd been gaining weight steadily since college, but it was really amplified after I had kids. I really wanted to do something, but I couldn't figure out what to do to get myself into a routine that would work for me. It also seemed like everything I was interested in had a high entry point, like I felt I would have to be in really good shape to even try the activities I found interesting.

"A friend had told me about Dustin's boot camps, so I signed up for three weeks last summer. I figured I could do anything for three weeks! I've stuck with it ever since. It's been a great life change. I feel like I just know so much more. I even think I'm mentally a little bit sharper because of being healthier. I feel so much better. I've got more energy, and I'm actually less tired at the end of the day now, even though I'm getting up at quarter to five in the morning. I'm wearing a size 8 or 10 now, which is great. I never pictured myself in the single digits!"

Tina's current goals: "I'm going to do some 5Ks. I want to continue to get stronger, and I definitely still have some problem areas or 'family inheritances' I'm working on. I have other people in my life who I know are interested but aren't sure they can do it, so I want to figure out a way to encourage them to take on the challenge."

Tina's advice to you: "Have a plan of some sort in mind, and have people who are going to hold you accountable for it. Share your plan and your goals with people. As much as you hope that you're going to be able to do it yourself, it is hard and you're going to have those moments when you're like, 'Can I do this? Is it really going to work for me?'"

Read more of Tina's story at *fitmomsforlife.com/tina.*

Tina, 36, mother of two. 5'6", 145 pounds. Tina lost more than 40 pounds in her first five months of coming to my boot camp.

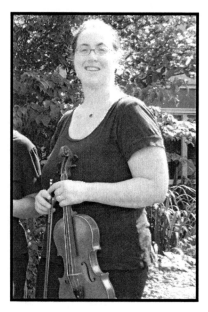

Goal Setting

In the last chapter, we talked about the importance of understanding your motivation and your reasons for wanting to get in shape. The next step in planning your fitness journey is to set the goals you want to accomplish. Do you want to run a marathon? Are you trying to drop two sizes to get back to your pre-baby clothes? Are you trying to lose fat before you have another child? Do you want to look great for a vacation, reunion, or wedding coming up? As my client Lynn put it, "Whether your goal is to do so many push-ups or to lose so many pounds or to be stronger, it gives you something to work toward. I don't think they ever have to end. You just have to keep making new goals."

A recent study by Gail Matthews, Ph.D., at Dominican University of California found that people who wrote down their goals for a four-week period made one and a half times as much progress toward accomplishing their goals as those who simply thought about their goals but did not write them down. The study also showed that people who told a friend about their goals made more progress than those who did not, and that those who provided a friend with weekly progress reports made even more progress. This study demonstrates the importance of writing down goals, making a public commitment to achieve your goals, and holding yourself accountable. So now it's time to determine where you want to go with your health and fitness, write down your goals, and get started accomplishing them.

The Importance of Goals

Like a ship in the sea, you need to know where you're going if you want to chart a course, stay on that course, and eventually reach your destination. Your goals are like the rudder of the ship. The rudder keeps the ship moving in the right direction as it passes through different currents and weather. With good goals in place, you'll be able to make decisions every day that keep you moving toward your destination and to resist temptations that could pull you off course.

Goals are also great from a measurement standpoint. As human beings, we like to see where we are today compared with a month ago or six months ago. In the next chapter, I'll guide you through tests and measurements that will help establish your baseline. Goals themselves are also a type of measurement. Three months from now, six months from now, you can look back at the goals you set today and see how many of them you've accomplished and how far you've come. If you aren't reaching your goals, that's an indication that you need to reassess what you're doing. Maybe you aren't putting in the effort you need to; maybe your goals were too ambitious. Either way, sitting down to reconsider your goals and your progress is a way to keep yourself on track.

I like to look back at my yearly goals for myself. On average I reach about 80 percent of them, and I usually find I've made progress toward the other ones as well. While I think you should set goals you can achieve (as I'm going to describe below), I know that different types of goals can be motivating, too. One of the trainers who worked with me, Joe Sweeney, is a huge goal setter and a positive thinker.

He recently challenged me to set monthly goals with him. Joe might set 10 goals for a month. Even if he only reaches two or three of them that month, he still knows he's further along in the other areas than he would have been if he hadn't set those goals. He operates on the idea that if you shoot for the moon and fall short, you'll still be among the stars.

> " Think of a goal for yourself—something that is going to motivate you to get out of bed in the morning and do your workout."
>
> – Jane

Other people take a different approach. My client Sandra started out with a weight-loss goal of 10 pounds. Once she reached it, she set a goal to lose another 10, and then another. She eventually lost 32 pounds, but by breaking it up into smaller chunks, she never felt overwhelmed and was able to celebrate her accomplishments along the way. Laura is another client who broke her goals down. "It can be overwhelming if you look at the whole picture," she explained. "Make it into smaller bundles so you can make those little steps."

How to Set Good Goals

The word to keep in mind as you're setting goals is SMART. Smart goals are Specific, Measurable, Attainable, Realistic, and Timed.[1] Use the chart on page 174 to write out your own goals that meet these criteria.

The biggest mistake I see people making when they're setting goals is that they make them too generic. If your goal is just "lose weight" or "feel better," how will you ever know whether you've reached it? Likewise, it needs to be measurable. There needs to be some concrete thing that will

---

1 Doran, G. T. "There's a S.M.A.R.T. Way to Write Management's Goals and Objectives." <u>Management Review </u>70.11 (1981): 35-36.

change if you reach your goal.

The next two aspects of a good goal are that it is attainable and realistic. Again, these go together. Setting big, pie-in-the-sky goals for yourself is fine if you find that motivating, but you need to have smaller ones too, so that you can see the progress you're making. You need some goals that are attainable—changes you can make within a reasonable time frame—so that you don't get discouraged along the way. Your goals also need to be realistic about what it's possible to accomplish, whether in a specific time frame or just in general.

Finally, a good goal is timed. Without a deadline, a goal is just something you'd like to do someday! Deadlines help keep you focused and accountable. The time frame you set will depend on what type of goal it is—some people set daily, weekly, monthly, and/or yearly goals, and some might be on an even longer time frame. You need to craft a goal that makes sense for the time frame you've chosen.

Let's use weight loss as an example. "I want to lose 15 pounds." This is a good start. It's a very specific goal, and it is definitely measurable. For the typical person, losing 15 pounds is attainable and realistic, given enough time. (Of course, if you weigh only 105 pounds to start with or are already very fit, it would be an unrealistic—not to mention unhealthy—goal!) You need a timetable for the goal, and you must remember to keep it attainable and realistic: "I want to lose 15 pounds in three months" or by a specific date.

"Feeling better" is another goal a lot of people have when they set out to improve their health and fitness. It takes a little more work to turn that into a specific, measurable goal. You need to come up with something more tangible, because "feeling better" can mean so many different things. You might say, "I want to have enough energy that I don't have to drink coffee at two o'clock in the afternoon to stay awake." You could say you want to achieve this goal within one month of starting my fitness program. Or "feeling better" might mean resolving pain or reducing your need for a certain medication. So your goal would be: "Within a month, I will reduce the ibuprofen I take for back pain each week by at least half."

One other thing about good goals is that they are visible! Maybe in the past you've taken the time to write out some goals, but then left them on your computer or inside a book and forgotten about them. I suggest you print your goals out or write them on sticky notes and put them where you can see them, so that you don't forget what you're working toward.

Thinking Short-Term and Long-Term

There are a lot of different theories about how many goals people should set and what time frames they should use. It can get overwhelming to have a huge number of goals. Personally, I like to set daily goals, one-week goals, one-month goals, six-month goals, and then some longer-term goals for what I want to achieve in one to 10 years.

For fitness, I think the most important goals are within that first year. My belief is that you could be in the best shape of your life—within 5 to 10 percent of your genetic potential—a year from now if you really commit to making the necessary changes. (If you're morbidly obese, you may need a couple of years to lose the excess weight.) Setting ambitious fitness-related goals for one year from now is a really good idea, but you probably also need to have shorter-term goals that will get you to that point.

A daily goal might be to drink 12 cups of water. That has all the attributes of a SMART goal. By setting that as a daily goal, you're committing to doing your best to achieve it every day. You'll need a way to track whether you reach it each day. You might have a large water bottle you need to fill four times, or you might keep a tally of the cups of water you drink. Somehow, you need to measure whether you reach that goal each day. If you don't drink much water now, you might want to work your way up to drinking that much—you might aim for six cups a day for one week, eight cups a day the next, and so on. Just don't make the mistake Jennifer made: She saw the advice to drink two to three liters of water a day, but she misread it and thought it said two to three gallons. Being very goal-oriented, she did it for a few days—and did nothing else besides running to the bathroom—before realizing her mistake!

As you get into weekly and monthly goals, you can start to look at weight lost or sizes lost. Strength goals are also great as monthly goals: "I'll be able to do five push-ups one month from today." Or, "I want to do a pull-up by three months from now."

Once you have set some goals, you also need to check back and adjust them, and set new ones occasionally. Of course, the shorter the time frame, the more often you should reassess. With yearly or longer-term goals, I'd suggest glancing at them every two or three months to see how you're doing and then adjust as needed.

Long-term physical goals are also important. Whether it is maintaining a certain body-fat percentage, running a certain number of miles each year, or just being injury-free, long-term goals can help balance out the short-term desires for weight loss or size loss and remind you of the bigger picture.

Setting Goals Beyond Physical Fitness

I highly recommend setting some goals for yourself that are not about your physical fitness, health, or weight loss. Of course, this book is about fitness, and that's my area of expertise. But setting goals and working toward them is something you can use to make changes and achieve your dreams in all areas of your life. When I set goals, they are not exclusively about fitness. I have goals for my business—like the goal I shared earlier, to reach one million moms by the end of 2015—and for my own professional development and personal life. I set goals to keep myself motivated, to stay on track, and to help track how much I've accomplished—not just physically, but in so many other ways—and I encourage you to do the same.

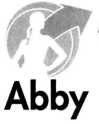

Fit Moms for Life Transformation

Abby

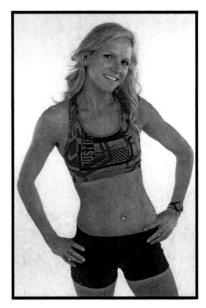

Abby has transformed her body and is now a personal trainer, boot camp instructor, and fitness model competitor. She is living proof that women can get very strong without bulking up—she can squat more weight than I can and can do 12 pull-ups, all while fitting into a size 2.

Abby's story: "Dustin always says that before I started his programs, I was the cardio queen. I would go to the gym for an hour to an hour and a half, four or five nights a week, and would use the elliptical machine and the treadmill. I wasn't burning many calories, and I wasn't working up much of a sweat. Unfortunately, I also wasn't seeing any results. I started going to Dustin's core class and doing small-group personal training with him, cutting back on the cardio—and that's when I started to see results.

"Right before I started training with Dustin I was about 150 pounds and over 25 percent body fat. My body was a little bit squishier than I would have liked. When I went from not lifting weights at all to lifting a lot, I actually put on a few pounds. But once I focused on nutrition and started paying attention to what I was putting into my body, the weight really started to come off.

*Abby, 27.
5'7", 128 pounds.
Abby gave up her "cardio queen"
habit and transformed her body,
losing almost 25 pounds in a year
and getting below 14 percent
body fat.*

"It took me about a year to lose 20 to 25 pounds. It was a slow process, and frustrating at times, but it was definitely worth it. I can't even begin to explain how happy I am that I stuck with it. I've become a lot more confident, and I have more faith in my ability to do something. I really learned that if I put my mind to it, I can accomplish anything."

Abby's exercise tips: "Get off the cardio equipment and get into the weight room! Total body weight training is the best way to build muscle and burn fat, so get in there and do that a few times a week. Add some high-intensity interval training two or three days a week, and you're going to see massive changes."

Abby's advice to you: "Have faith in yourself, believe in yourself, and know that you're worth it! Now, go out and do something about it!"

Read more of Abby's story at *fitmomsforlife.com/abby.*

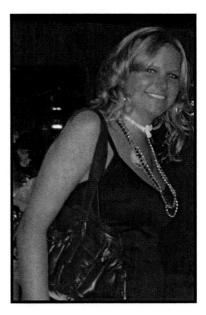

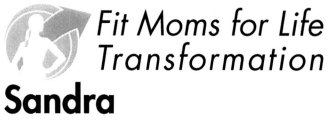

Fit Moms for Life Transformation
Sandra

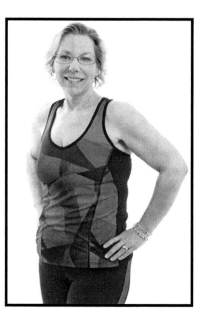

Sandra has seen amazing results using the *Fit Moms for Life* and *Got Core* DVDs, and weighs less now than she did when she got married.

Sandra's story: "I had gained weight after each of my kids—common story. About five years ago, I actually lost 70 pounds mostly just by dieting and walking. I was really excited about that, and happy with it. But life gets in the way sometimes, and I ended up gaining about 35 pounds back. Last summer I saw a picture of myself and was appalled at how I had let myself go. At the time I was 48, so I decided to set some personal goals for my career, family, and health as I looked ahead to turning 50. I started using Dustin's DVDs religiously, three days a week, and focused on lifestyle changes. I'm really focusing on making this transformation for myself for the long term. I'm looking at my health and making an investment in myself so that I can be active for another 50 years.

"I've lost the weight that I had put back on, and I feel great. Last time, I got down to 144 pounds and was in a size 14. Now that I'm focusing on strength training, I'm in a size 6 at 138 pounds. I've also found that with all the strength training and all the focus on the core, I don't have the problems with my back that I had in the past. I love how I feel at a healthy weight and being active. I encourage my friends and family to work out with me.

"My husband and family are incredibly proud of me. Even my 15-year-old is like, 'Mom, good for you. I'm really proud you that you're sticking with this and you're working out.'"

Sandra's current goals: "I'm hoping to do a 100K (61-mile) bike ride in May. In addition, I have set goals around many aspects of my life, including career, personal growth, and family."

Read more of Sandra's story at *fitmomsforlife.com/sandra*.

Sandra, 49, mother of three. 5'2", 138 pounds. Sandra discovered strength training in the Fit Moms for Life DVDs and has toned up and lost more than 40 pounds.

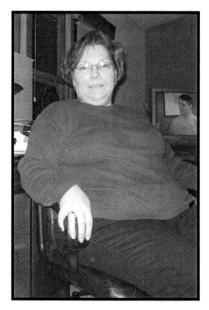

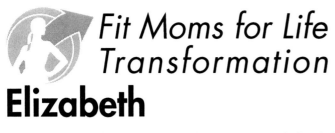

Fit Moms for Life Transformation

Elizabeth

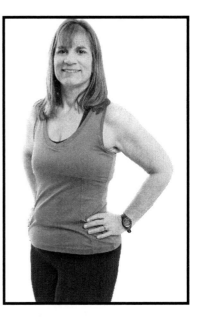

Elizabeth got off the dieting roller coaster and decided to make sustainable changes in her life. She's been coming to my boot camps for a year now and has made great progress with weight loss, increased strength, and improved self-confidence.

Elizabeth's story: "A little over a year ago, I went to see my nurse practitioner and she told me I weighed more than I had when I was nine months pregnant with my daughter—close to 200 pounds. That was kind of a wake-up call. That same week, my daughter told me I wasn't the fattest mom in her kindergarten class—there was one mom who was fatter than I was. She thought she was being kind.

"I had lost weight many times before, but I wanted to do it differently this time. For the first time, I was looking at my health instead of looking at fitting into a certain size or getting skinny for a wedding, my own or somebody else's. And I really looked at what kind of role model I was going to be for my daughter. I probably could have had my food delivered to me or been on some really wacky low-calorie diet. It would work for a while, and I'd lose weight. But it wouldn't be sustainable. And it would tell my daughter that you should be in a fight with your body. I didn't want it to be a battle with food and exercise. It should be about feeling good.

Elizabeth, 46, mother of one. 5'4", 143 pounds. Elizabeth lost 47 pounds and got down to a size 6 within a year of starting my program.

"Now, after a year of Dustin's boot camps, I've lost 47 pounds. I can do things now I couldn't have done a year ago. I've also taken a job with more management responsibilities and started to see myself as a leader. I think success breeds success. If you're successful in one area of your life, you're like, 'I can do this.'"

Elizabeth's nutrition tips: "I used to be kind of an all-or-nothing person. I think goal-directed people tend to be. It's like, 'I have to be perfect or skip the whole thing.' And I've learned I can still eat some things that probably aren't the best, but then I just look at cutting back a little bit the next day. It's not all-or-nothing anymore. It is more about the whole package."

Read more of Elizabeth's story at *fitmomsforlife.com/elizabeth.*

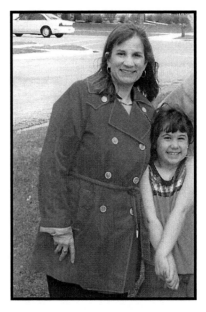

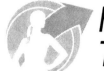

Fit Moms for Life Transformation

Laura

Laura is my "slow and steady wins the race" client. She has made a gradual transformation by doing what was within her abilities and is seeing amazing results.

Laura's story: "I've battled with being overweight a good portion of my life. I had a serious neck injury about six years ago and had to have surgery. That caused some general health issues, and I had core muscle issues and really, really bad core strength. Just going down the steps carrying a basket of laundry felt like a lot of work. I felt like I couldn't even chase after my son if he were to run out into the street. It had gotten to be a quality-of-life issue. I just wasn't able to do everything I needed and wanted to do.

"To start with, my goal was getting to MamaTone three times a week. It was just the mental aspect of getting myself there and realizing it was something I had to do. I lost 10 pounds and gained strength and endurance just doing the exercise. But then it finally clicked that you can't just eat whatever you want all the time, and I changed my eating habits, and that really brought the weight off.

"After 18 months of MamaTone, I'm the strongest I've ever been, I feel better, I've gone from a size 22 to size 14, and I weigh about what I did in high school. When I started, I could only go three to four miles per hour on the treadmill. Now I can do sprints at over nine miles per hour. It feels awesome to be able to do that, with all the other moms around me going, 'Rock on!'

"In general, I feel more confident about myself. I always tell my kids that they can do anything they set their mind to. And it finally clicked in my own brain that I can do that too."

Laura's advice to you: "If you are where I was—242 pounds and physically limited—something isn't working. You need to realize that you have to make some changes, inform yourself, and start to push those boundaries. You just have to do it in a way that's going to work for you."

Read more of Laura's story at *fitmomsforlife.com/laura.*

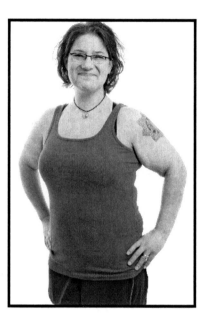

Laura, 38, mother of two. 5'5", 192 pounds. Laura has lost over 50 pounds and made incredible gains in flexibility, agility, and strength over the past 18 months.

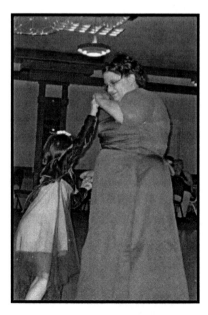

Getting Real

Are you ready to begin transforming your body and your life? There's one more important thing to do, either before you start or shortly after, and that is to get real and assess where you're starting from. We've talked about the importance of knowing where you want to go. Now let's talk about documenting where you are right now, so that you'll be able to see your progress over time.

Assess Where You're Starting From

I'm going to guide you through how to assess your current size, physical fitness, nutritional habits, and lifestyle. While some of these reality checks may seem painful right now, you will be grateful for them later. If you follow my program and make the changes I recommend, I guarantee you will see improvement in one or more of these areas. Many of the clients I interviewed for the transformation stories you see in this book told me they had to guess at their starting weight, that they had no idea how many inches they'd lost around their waists, and that they knew their first workouts were very challenging but didn't have any numbers to compare their abilities now to their abilities then. Of course, they're still proud of what they've accomplished, but they all wish they had taken the measurements, stood on the scale, and timed and tested themselves so that they could quantify the changes. They wish they had taken real "before" pictures that showed their starting point. So document it now and know you're setting out on a path to make changes in all of these areas.

> " Not taking measurements when I started is the biggest regret I have."
>
> – Crystal

If you're dreading weighing yourself, taking body measurements, or making a realistic assessment of your fitness and nutrition levels, that might be a sign you're in denial. A lot of people are. Many of my clients look back at their "before" pictures, after they've lost a lot of weight, and don't even recognize the person in the picture. They never accepted that they had gotten as big as they had. They were in denial about how bad it had gotten, because it happened gradually over time, and they stopped really looking in the mirror at some point. Every picture they saw of themselves was "taken from a bad angle." Maybe this sounds familiar to you. If it does, it's time to get real.

I asked Marsue what moment started her on her journey toward losing more than 70 pounds of fat and becoming a personal trainer; she said she'd been watching her daughter's class at a karate studio. "Looking at my reflection in the mirrors across the room, I didn't even recognize myself anymore," she said. "I knew I was unhappy. I just wasn't taking the steps." That was the moment that changed her life!

A lot of people also have an unrealistic estimation of their own abilities, which often goes hand in hand with being in denial. I've seen this go both directions. When some people come to my classes for the first time, they think they're in great shape, and they just get destroyed

> **"** The first step is to realize that the picture is not lying to you."
>
> – Lynda

by the class. They realize that the type of exercise they've been doing hasn't been making them fit or that their sense of what they can do is rooted in the past, before they put on 20 pounds or back when they used to work out every day in college.

More often, though, I see women who go the other way and don't give themselves enough credit. They don't think they can handle the workout. They don't think they can do a push-up. They don't think they can run a sprint for 30 seconds. And maybe they can't do all of those things the first time they try, but they can almost always do more than they thought they could. As they gain strength, lose weight, and develop the confidence to try new things, they find out they can do all of them and more. Doing the fitness assessment I'm recommending here will give you a realistic sense of what you can do now and what potential you have for improvement.

Another reason I'm asking you to document where you are right now in so many areas is that there will be times you make progress in one area but not another. People tend to focus just on their weight on the scale, but there may be weeks where that number doesn't budge. (If you're doing intensive strength training and are not changing your eating, or if you're starting at a healthy weight and adding muscle, that number might even go up.) If that's all you're looking at, you might get discouraged and be tempted to throw in the towel. Having a lot of different measurements can keep you going during those times when you're not feeling good about yourself. You might not have lost any weight, but you took an inch off your waist in the past month. Maybe you've increased how long you can hold a plank by a full minute since you started. Or perhaps you can run at a high speed for

30 seconds now, compared with just 10 seconds two months ago. When you can see that progress, you're going to feel more motivated to keep up the hard work, tweak your efforts as needed, and get to the results you want to see overall.

Baseline measurements are also the key to setting realistic goals and tracking progress toward them. Let's say you want to be able to do 50 push-ups. You need to know your starting point, not just to track changes over time, but also so that you can set a realistic goal. Your goal will be very different if you can only do five push-ups today than if you're starting out at 25. Your starting point will help you determine how long you should give yourself to reach your goal—and whether you need to set some shorter-term goals along the way.

Physical Reality Check

Pictures. Taking "before" and "after" pictures is one of the most powerful things you can do to document your progress. You've got to do this. If I started my career over again, I would personally take a picture of every one of my clients when they walked in the door on the first day, because so many people don't do it.

You can go to *fitmomsforlife.com/pictures* to see videos about how to take good pictures, but here are my basic tips:

For good pictures, you don't want to be wearing too many clothes. A swimsuit is what I usually recommend. (You can take naked pictures if you want to, but you probably aren't going to share those with many people. So for my sake, if you want to share your story with me as you get results, at least be wearing a swimsuit!) Shorts and a sports bra are also a good option for women, while others prefer bra and underwear.

Stand in front of a light background that is not too busy. You should take one picture from the front, one from the side, and one from the back. If you want to do the classic unhappy face, sticking out your belly and rounding your shoulders for the before picture, that's fine. Those make for good dramatic before and after pictures, but you should also take some more real ones where you're smiling and trying to look your best.

I recommend retaking your photos once a month, keeping everything as consistent as possible. Try to have the same background, the same lighting, and the camera the same distance away. Wear the same clothes—or the same style of clothes in a smaller size, as you go. You'll be able to start to see where your body is changing and where it's not changing.

Circumference measurements. The next thing to do is to take circumference measurements of some of the body parts that will change as you tone up and lose weight. I have videos about how to do this at *fitmomsforlife.com/measurements*, but here are the basics:

Wear very little clothing when taking body measurements, just as you did for your photos. You can do the measurements naked if you want, or you can wear thin clothes. The most important thing is to be consistent about what you are wearing each time you take measurements, so that the numbers aren't skewed from one time to the next. You'll be able to take most of these measurements yourself using a tape measure, but there are a couple you might need someone's help with. Don't flex your muscles or suck in your belly as you do these—just stay relaxed and keep breathing to get accurate measurements.

Here are the measurements I recommend you take, and some tips for how to get each one. (Note: On page 175, you can record each of these measurements today and over time.)

- **Chest:** For women, I recommend taking two measurements. First, measure along your bra band at the top of your rib cage. Then measure again going around your breasts while wearing a bra. (For better or for worse, your cup size—which is based on the difference between these two measurements—is probably going to go down as you lose body fat.)
- **Waist:** The waist is actually defined as the skinniest part of your torso, most likely above your belly button. Try bending side to side, and see where you bend—that's going to be your skinniest part and where you want to measure.
- **Abdomen:** You want an additional measurement in your abdomen, ideally around the fattest part. Depending on your body type, that may be higher or lower. I usually try to go approximately around the belly button and include the love-handle area for this measurement.
- **Hips:** The hips are the basically the biggest part of the butt. Measure around the largest area, keeping the tape measure parallel to the floor.
- **Thigh:** This one is a little tricky, because you have to be sure to measure the same spot on your thigh each time. I suggest you find the midpoint between your knee and your hip joint, and measure there.
- **Arm:** Just like with the thigh, it's important to measure the same spot on your arm each time. Find the midpoint between your shoulder joint and your elbow, and measure around.

Weight. Weighing yourself is kind of a given, even though I advise people not to focus too much on the scale for a variety of reasons. As I've said before, your weight might go up as you build muscle, especially if you aren't losing fat at the same time (which could be because you don't have a lot of fat to lose or because you aren't changing your eating habits). I've seen women gain between four and eight pounds of muscle in a six-month period, and if you aren't losing fat to make up for that, your weight will go up. In general, the closer you are to your ideal weight, the less you should pay attention to your weight as an indicator of your progress. That said, weight is still an important measurement, and it is a simple one to take and track over time.

Stepping on a scale can be very emotional for some people. If you attach too much meaning to the number on it, then you should cut back on how often you weigh yourself and focus more on body measurements, strength gains, and how your clothes feel. But even if it is difficult, I would really encourage you to at least take a starting weight, so that in six months you can look back and know how much you've lost.

If you're able to be unemotional about it, I recommend weighing yourself once a day—first thing in the morning, after you've gone to the bathroom, without any clothes on. Your weight will go up and down somewhat, depending on factors such as how hydrated you are and where you are in your menstrual cycle. At the end of each week, take the average of all the weights you recorded that week, and consider that your weight for the week. That will give you a more accurate sense of the direction you're going than if you just step on the scale once a week or once a month. It should also help you from going into an emotional tailspin if your weight is up half a pound one morning. Just remind yourself that you are going to average it in with your other weigh-ins from the week, and then it's not as big a deal.

Body-fat percentage. This isn't really something you can measure on your own, but if you have access to a qualified trainer, it's a great measurement to get. Most gyms and Y facilities will provide this service for a small fee. Get it measured now, and do it again in six months to see how much you've lost. (Home scales that measure body-fat percentage are pretty inaccurate. I'd rather see you put that money toward exercise equipment or high-quality food. If you do use one of those scales, just try to be really consistent about the time of day you weigh yourself, your body temperature, and hydration level. You should be able to see change over time, even if the percentage it's giving you isn't that accurate.)

Fitness Reality Check

The next step is to assess your current fitness level. These tests will show you where you're at and will establish a baseline for comparison over time. You may be familiar with some of these exercises already. For those exercises you are unfamiliar with, check out the demonstrations at *fitmomsforlife. com/testing* in addition to the photos here, to be sure you're doing them right.

I recommend getting into comfortable clothes and running shoes and warming up before doing these tests. (See pages 121-123 for a sample warm-up.) If you haven't been exercising a lot lately, consider these tests the first workout on your journey! Do the tests and then, if you have the energy, do more of the exercises in Chapter 9. If you already have an exercise routine in place, do these tests after warming up but before you've worked hard, so that you can give these your all. You will need a carpeted floor or yoga mat, as well as a wall you can sit against. Have a stopwatch handy or a clock

> " I remember trying to do my first plank and hardly lasting 10 or 15 seconds. Even though that first day was so hard, just having that little bit of success, you kind of thrive on feeling good about what you did, and it keeps you coming back."
> – Liz

with a second hand in sight, so that you can time yourself on several of these tests. Write down on page 176 how long you could hold the exercise or how many reps you were able to do. The table on page 42 shows you where your performance falls compared to other women and may help you set goals for improvement.

Retest yourself about once a month and track improvements. This is a great way to identify where you're doing well and areas where you need to focus more. Another thing I really like about doing these tests is that if you're following my exercise program, you're going to see improvements. Even if you're eating too much, or the wrong things, and even if you're not strength

> *When I started with Dustin, I couldn't do a single push-up. And now I can do 50 toe push-ups without stopping, which still impresses me."*
>
> – Vanessa

training hard, you'll get fitter and improvements will show up in these tests. It's almost physiologically impossible not to get better when you're training your body this way. This is one area in which all of my clients see results, even when they aren't losing weight, and that progress can keep you going through the tough times.

Front plank. Place your forearms on the ground with your shoulders positioned right above your elbows. Toes are on the ground. The abs are drawn in and the legs are contracted. Hold this position while breathing naturally. Make sure your hips don't stick up too high or sag too low. If your lower back starts to bother you, or your back starts to sag or arch, that's when you need to stop. Write down how long you were able to hold it.

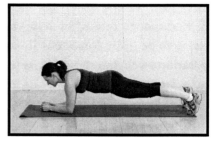

Push-ups. Everyone knows what a push-up is, but a lot of people do them with poor form. To do a good push-up, place your hands wider than your shoulders but in line with the shoulders and chest. Lower your chest toward the ground, stopping when your shoulder is at the same height as your elbow. Make sure to keep your abs pulled in, and maintain neutral alignment throughout the exercise. (Neutral alignment is the natural curvature the spine should adopt when you are standing straight up. There should be a natural curve in your lower back.) Do as many push-ups on your toes as you are able to—this is called working to failure. By the way, I don't consider knee push-ups to be actual push-ups. If you're unable to do even one push-up on your toes, then you can go down to your knees and do them, again keeping

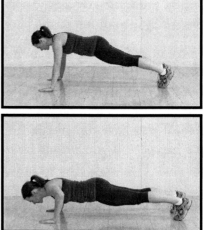

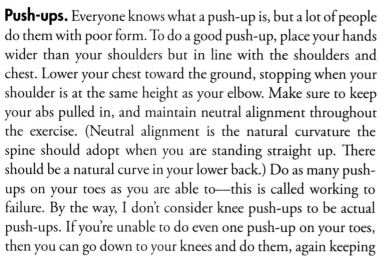

your hands under your chest and shoulder area and keeping your back flat. Note on page 176 how many you did. If you did them on your knees, note that.

Burpees. To do a burpee, start from a standing position. Jump up with your hands above your head. Then drop down to a push-up position and bring your chest to the ground. Then take your hands and bring them down to your sides with the palms up. Once you do that, bring your hands forward again to support you, bring your feet forward, and jump up as quickly as possible. That is one rep. Keep your form consistent, doing as many as you can in 90 seconds. Write down your number of reps.

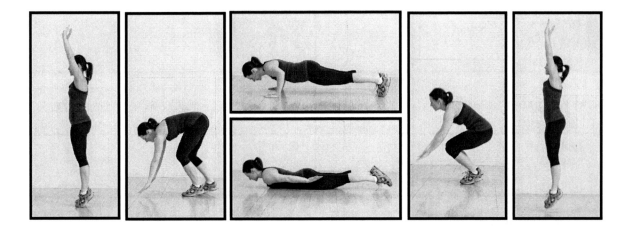

Wall sit. Find a wall and sit back onto it. Lower yourself so that your thighs are parallel to the ground and your knees are right over your heels. Let your arms hang at your sides. While timing yourself, hold that position for as long as you can; mark down your time. Your legs will be burning! If you're already in good shape, this is going to be pretty easy for you. If you're already in the "Above average" or "Superstar" category, you may want to hold some dumbbells by your side to make it more difficult (and, of course, mark down the weight of the dumbbells).

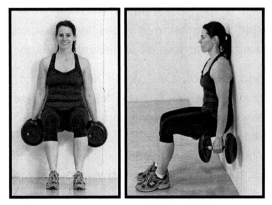

Cardiovascular endurance. Finally, I want you to test your cardiovascular endurance. You are going to time yourself running or walking as fast as you can for a mile. Whether you do this on a treadmill, track, or road, make sure to use the same location for your retests. By the end of a mile, you should have pushed yourself to your max and be completely exhausted. Note on page 176 where you ran or walked, and how long it took you.

Benchmarks: Fitness Tests

Test	Biggest need for improvement	Below average	Average	Above average	Superstar
Front plank (seconds)	1-20	20-40	40-60	60-120	120+
Push-ups (reps)	0	1-5	5-10	10-30	30+
Burpees (reps in 90 seconds)	1-10	11-17	18-25	25-30	30+
Wall sit, no weights (seconds)	1-30	30-60	60-120	120-180	180+
Mile run or walk (minutes)	>12	10-12	8-10	7-8	<7

Nutritional Reality Check

Getting real about nutrition is a huge part of figuring out what it's going to take to get in the best shape of your life. You need to take a good hard look at what you are putting into your body. At this point, I'm not asking you to change how you eat, just to assess and document what you're currently eating, so that you can identify the changes you want to make and start implementing them.

Food journal. One of the most powerful tools for weight loss is a food journal. You've probably heard this before, but very few people have actually ever kept one. The main idea is to write down everything you eat for a period of five to seven days. (You don't have to do a full week, but you do need to include a weekend, because people tend to eat very differently on the weekends.) It's going to be a little painful, and it's going to be tedious, but luckily there are some great technological tools that can do a lot of the work for you.

Each day for those five to seven days, write down every single thing you eat and drink, including the portion size. I recommend you buy a digital food scale to do this accurately—at about $30 for a cheap one, it's one of the best investments you can make for the sake of nutrition, and it will come in handy later as you work to improve your eating, too. This way, you will be able to determine how many calories you're eating based on exactly how much food you ate. You can use the food journal form on page 177. (Photocopy that page, or download the blank form at *fitmomsforlife.com/foodjournal*.)

Use nutrition labels on food to determine how many calories and grams of carbs, fats, and protein are in everything you eat and drink. This is also where technology comes into play. Using a website such as CalorieKing or Livestrong, or a nutritional values reference book available at most libraries, you can look up almost any brand-name packaged food, restaurant meal, or natural food (like an apple) and find the calories, carbs, fats, and protein in it. Websites like *sparkpeople.com* and *loseit.com* and smartphone apps like Lose It! and Calorie Tracker actually allow you to keep an electronic food journal where all those values are calculated; this can save you a lot of time. It still gets tedious entering every single thing you eat and drink—but remember, it's only for a week. My recommendation is that you write down what you eat in a small notebook you can carry with you, and then look up all the amounts or enter everything into an online food journal at once when you have a chance later.

> " When I wrote down how much stuff I ate in a day, I was shocked."
>
> – Patty H.

It is important to be accurate in your recording and to measure your portion sizes. People tend to underestimate how many calories they eat, especially with larger meals. A study in 2006 found that people estimated the calories in a small fast food meal fairly accurately, but underestimated the calories in large meals by an average of 22 percent.[1] In that study, overweight people were more likely to have eaten larger meals and therefore more likely to underestimate the calories they were consuming. Overweight people underestimated their calorie intake by an average of 33 percent, compared with an average underestimate of 16 percent among people of a healthy weight. That means that when those overweight people thought a meal contained 600 calories, they were actually eating 800 calories. A difference like that adds up to a lot over the course of a day!

After the week is over, your food journal will help you answer the following questions:

- How many calories do you eat per day, on average? (See the box on page 44 to figure out how many calories you should be eating.)
- Did you eat a lot more some days than others? What was going on those days?
- What is the breakdown of carbs, fats, and proteins in your diet?
- How many times do you eat each day? At what times? Are you skipping breakfast? Are you just eating a few big meals, grazing all day, or doing something in between?
- How often are you snacking, and what do you eat when you snack?
- How many fruits and vegetables do you eat?
- Is there a certain time of day you tend to eat foods that aren't good for you?
- How often are you eating out?
- Are there things in your food journal you wouldn't want your kids to eat? Are there things you wouldn't want your kids (or husband or friends) to know you're eating?

---

1 Wansink, B., and P. Chandon. "Meal Size, Not Body Size, Explains Errors in Estimating the Calorie Content of Meals." Annals of Internal Medicine 145 (2006): 326-32.

A few other questions you can ask yourself for your nutritional reality check are:

- How often do you grocery shop?
- Do you buy a lot of fresh fruits and vegetables?
- Do you buy a lot of processed foods?
- How much time do you spend on food preparation each week?
- What do you feed your kids? Do they eat the same foods as you, or are you a short-order cook making a separate meal for everyone in the family?

How Many Calories Do You Need?

I can't tell you exactly how many calories you need to eat to lose weight, because that's going to differ for everyone. I've found that 1,500 calories per day or fewer works for weight loss for most women, and around 2,000 calories is good for men. I definitely don't like to see anyone go lower than 1,200 calories per day, because then your metabolism starts to slow down to save energy, and long-term weight loss and maintenance are very hard to achieve.

As a starting point, if you're a woman and weight loss is one of your goals, aim to stay below 1,500 calories per day. If you're trying to maintain your current weight, try to consume between 1,500 and 2,000 calories a day. Anything above 2,000 calories per day will likely cause you to gain weight, unless you're working out intensely for at least an hour a day. More than 2,500 calories a day will almost certainly cause weight gain.

Self-Care Reality Check

The final piece of this reality check is to take a comprehensive look at how well you are taking care of your whole self. So many moms don't take care of themselves as well as they take care of others. In the long run, that isn't going to benefit anyone! As I've said before, you need to take care of yourself so that you will have the energy and ability to take care of others. Remember, put your own oxygen mask on first! You may already have had some insights into these issues as you read Chapter 2 about mindset, but now I want you to think about how well you are doing in each of these areas as you begin this transformation.

Time for yourself. This is where so many moms struggle. Whether you are home with kids full time or juggling work and family responsibilities, it is hard to get time to yourself while your kids are growing up. I think every mom should set aside 30 to 45 minutes every day, at least five days a week, for "mom time."

I know this can be difficult if you're a single mom or your husband works long hours and you're home alone with kids a lot of the time. Maybe you don't have family or friends nearby who can help take care of your kids. But if at all possible, try to carve out that time for yourself. Maybe you can find time when the kids are napping or in the early morning before they get up. Or join a gym that offers child care, so that you can work out a few times a week while the kids play. Just take some time for yourself to exercise, to plan your healthy meals, or to relax with a good book or your favorite TV show.

Sleep. If you are not getting enough sleep, it's hard to have the energy to take care of everything you need to. Sleep is also very important for your health, as your body needs that time to recover from the day's activities, repair itself, and renew. Eight hours of sleep every night is ideal. Seven hours is pretty good. Getting six hours or less for an extended period of time can increase your levels of cortisol, the stress hormone, and that can help pack on the pounds.[2] Using that "mom time" for a nap is totally okay, too—especially if you're not getting good sleep at night because you have a baby or a sick child. My client

> " *I was the last person to take time for myself—even when I was exercising, it was with my kids in the jogging stroller. Getting up at five or 5:30 in the morning to do this while they're sleeping is not easy. And it takes a little commitment, but every time I thank myself when I'm done, because I feel so much better."*
>
> – Karen E.

Nancy realized that not getting enough sleep was keeping her from breaking through a weight-loss plateau. Once she had figured that out, she began heading to bed earlier. As she put it, "Nothing great happens after 10:30 at night anyway, so you might as well just go to bed." Once she started getting enough sleep, she got back on track with her weight loss.

Exercise patterns. How many days a week are you making time to exercise? How long are you exercising each time? How intense are your workouts? Are you doing cardio, strength training, or both?

Think about how much time you spend on exercise and what you get out of it. If you aren't exercising at all right now, or you aren't doing any intense workouts, making time for that is going to be your first step. If you're already working out, I bet you're going to find that my program takes less of your time and gets you greater results. Give it your full effort and see what you can accomplish.

With my program, even if you only have 15 minutes to exercise on some days, if you push yourself and do something intense for those 15 minutes, it can still be pretty powerful. Remind yourself that doing something is better than doing nothing, and make it as effective as you can. Or if you have chunks of time—say, 10 minutes a couple times during the day—you can break the workout into sections. But ideally, you'd take about 30 to 45 minutes for exercise. There's really no need to work out more than an hour at any given time, unless you're training for something like a marathon.

---

2 Knutson, Kristen L., and Eve Van Cauter. "Associations between Sleep Loss and Increased Risk of Obesity and Diabetes." <u>Annals of the New York Academy of Sciences</u> 1129.1 (2008): 287-304.

Attitude toward exercise. I meet some women who despise exercise. They really hate it, and no amount of coaxing and convincing is going to change their minds. If you can relate to this, I have some tips for you. As long as you hate exercise, it's going to be a challenge to do it consistently. So take a minute to write down the reasons you know exercise is good for you and the benefits you will glean from it. Next, I want you to write down some positive affirmations proclaiming the joys of exercise and the many benefits exercise will add to your life. Say these affirmations throughout the day. For example, "I enjoy the feeling I get from exercise when I sweat and my heart pumps fast. It is great knowing that I am becoming healthier, my bones are getting denser, my muscles are getting more toned, and my heart is getting stronger. I love exercise and will continue to do it for the rest of my life." I'm willing to bet that a person who uses affirmations like that is more likely to stick with a program than someone with a sourpuss attitude.

My client Aimee is a great example of someone who turned around her attitude toward exercise. Aimee hated me and my program the first time she tried it. She still claims to hate cardio, even in small doses, but she has come to love lifting heavy weights—she even asks for heavier weights a lot of the time! Most important, she's gotten past her negative attitude to make exercise part of her daily routine. "I get up, I get dressed, and I go to MamaTone," she told me. "There's no negotiating in the parking lot, which I used to do. Like, 'Maybe I should go to Target...' This is just part of my day now."

Taking It Too Far

Unfortunately, our culture pushes many people, especially women, to become unhealthily obsessed with food and exercise and being thin. I know I only see the tip of the iceberg, but I've still seen a lot of it in my work at fitness centers and as a personal trainer. I'm not a psychologist or a doctor, and I don't claim to understand everything women go through mentally, emotionally, and physically. But I have seen enough of this sort of unhealthy obsession to know what it looks like.

The warning signs that you might have a problem include:

Too much exercise. I think if you're working out more than an hour a day, six days a week, that's probably too much exercise. I'm not talking about working out in the morning and then going for a bike ride with your kids later in the day, and just having an active lifestyle. I'm talking about people who spend three to four hours a day on different cardio machines or who are constantly thinking about how many more calories they need to burn today. (Of course, some athletes train more than this to prepare for a marathon or Ironman triathlon. I would say if you're doing that or any other excessive exercise with the goal of burning calories, and it isn't a level of activity you can sustain in the long term, you may be taking it too far.)

Obsession with the scale. I see a lot of women who are emotionally tied to the number on the scale. The number on the scale in the morning determines their mood for the day. That's dangerous and unhealthy. We've already talked about the fact that the scale is only one part of the equation. But more important, the number on the scale doesn't define who you are. Obsession with the scale can be the first step in the cycle toward anorexia.

Obsession with the mirror. This is very similar to obsession with the scale. This is when you're always looking at yourself in the mirror and pointing out your flaws. Your butt is too big or your love handles are hanging over. Your thighs are rubbing together. Everyone has things they'd like to change about their body, but if you have a negative thought every time you look at your reflection, that's a bad sign.

Counting every calorie. Now this may sound odd, because I just told you to count calories when you do your food journal. But that's for a week, or every once in a while to see how you're doing and to stay realistic about what you're eating. Here I'm talking about obsessing over every single calorie you eat. I see this in many women who have a healthy body weight already. Of course, this leads to them adopting a severely restricted diet. When you start thinking of food as something to avoid, instead of as an energy source and a pleasurable experience, you're in the danger zone. When you freak out and search online to see how many calories the two pieces of celery you just ate contain, you probably have some issues to resolve.

Constantly thinking about weight loss, food, and/or exercise. The common thread is that you're constantly analyzing and thinking about your body in a negative way, through a constant internal dialogue. Looking good is great, but obsessing about it and overanalyzing it is not healthy and not what it's all about.

In my work as a trainer and running boot camps, I've seen many women get into what I'd call a negative cycle. They're doing the exercise part of my program, but they're afraid to give their bodies the fuel they need to support that kind of work. They can't handle eating four, five, or six times a day, so they either make their portions way too small or they skip meals and only eat a couple of times a day. They're also afraid to give up their long cardio workouts, so they keep doing hours on the treadmill. They really don't listen to my advice about eating a lot of protein and a decent amount of fat, so they're living on salads and trying to do a really intense workout program without enough fuel. If they're already at a healthy weight and they put on a couple of pounds with strength training, that freaks them out, so they cut back on their food even further. They can't eat the cheat meals that I recommend because it is so hard for them to take a break from counting calories, and their bodies are in starvation mode.

The bottom line is: You shouldn't be obsessed with your weight, your exercise, or your food in a way that makes it impossible for you to enjoy life. If you feel like this is an issue for you, find a specialist or a support group that specializes in body-image distortion issues or eating issues or over-exercise issues. If you don't know where to get help, talk to your doctor or call 2-1-1 for referrals to services in your community.

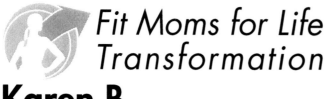

Fit Moms for Life Transformation

Karen B.

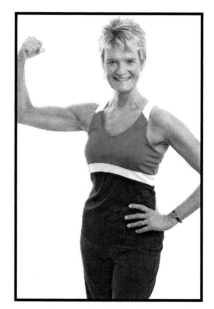

When I first met Karen, she was tall and thin with very little muscle tone—she looked frail to me, really. Two years later, she is an incredibly toned and lean postmenopausal woman determined to live life on her terms.

Karen's story: "I have always enjoyed being active, but it was nothing consistent. Then Dustin came to my home for a one-time personal training session about two years ago, and I haven't looked back. It has become a way of life for me. I got the 12 *Fit Moms for Life* DVDs, plus *Got Core* and *Buns, Guns, Back & Shoulders.* I mix and match to put together my workouts. I don't lift the same weights some of the younger mothers do in the DVDs, but I have made significant progress just by using the weights that are challenging for me. I feel empowered when I lift weights, and I like the change in my body. I feel good in body, mind, and spirit.

Karen B., 54, empty-nest mother of two. 5'7", 128 pounds. Karen gained eight pounds but stayed a size 6 as she gained strength and toned her body working out at home with my DVDs.

"I overcame an eating disorder in my younger days. As a result, I'm currently working with a nutritionist to better educate myself on how to eat to fuel my body to meet my nutritional needs, along with maintaining a healthy and fit lifestyle. I know I have to eat to get what I want as far as building muscle, strength, and endurance. I am gaining a new respect for my body and how it relates to nutrition, strength training, and cardio workouts. It's all about a fit lifestyle, and I will never go back!"

Karen's current goals: Karen recently achieved her dream of becoming an ACE-certified personal trainer. She wants to share her love and passion for health and fitness with others.

Read more of Karen's story at *fitmomsforlife.com/karenb.*

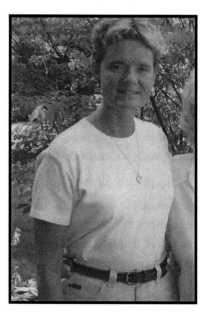

Fit Moms for Life Transformation

Liz

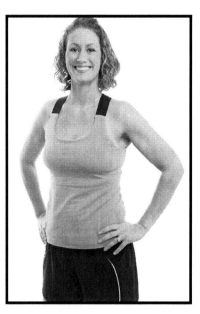

Liz has made a gradual but very effective transformation both physically and in terms of her outlook on life.

Liz's story: "I was a runner in high school, but I got injured and I pretty much let that take me down. For the next 10 years I didn't exercise and didn't eat exceptionally well. I suffered from a lot of depression through those years. I was on medication a couple of times for it.

"The day I got on the scale and saw the number 203, I sat down on the bathroom floor and cried. I was really disappointed in myself that I had let myself get to that point, and really upset that I wasn't being a role model for my children. That was an awful moment, but also a great moment, because it got me to where I am now. I started walking with a neighbor, and a few months later I started going to Dustin's MamaTone class.

"Now I'm proud of myself when I look in the mirror. This may be the first time in my life where I can honestly say that. I know I still have a little ways to go, but I have the strength and agility now to do the things I want to. Being able to really play with my kids has been a huge change for me. I've found happiness that I hadn't had in a long time."

Liz's current goals: "I'd like to lose another eight pounds and to run another marathon, and do it in closer to four hours."

Liz's nutrition tips: "Planning is the number one thing for me. On Sundays I sit down and look at what food came from our CSA or what food I froze from the garden, and make our menu for the week. And I make my grocery list based on that. If I just take that half hour Sunday night to plan everything, it's easy. You're not coming home trying to figure out what you're going to eat that night."

Read more of Liz's story at *fitmomsforlife.com/liz.*

Liz, 30, mother of two. 5'8", 148 pounds. Liz lost 55 pounds with my program in the last year and a half.

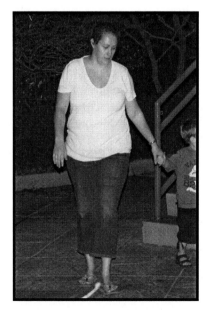

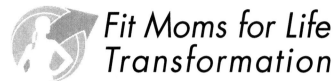

Fit Moms for Life Transformation

Jenny

Jenny had gradually put on weight over the years, but was able to drop it pretty quickly despite her busy schedule raising three kids with her husband and working as a nurse.

Jenny's story: "When I was in my twenties, I must have had a higher metabolism, because I would maintain my weight even if I didn't exercise. I never watched what I ate. But at some point everything just slowed down, and the weight packed on. I reached 198 pounds. On the BMI chart, I was considered obese and had high cholesterol.

"Working as a nurse, I've seen many, many health problems that can be avoided if people live healthier lives. I knew it was time to change my habits. I didn't want to go on meds for high cholesterol, so I finally started working out. I'm striving to live a better and healthier life so I can live life to the fullest.

"I've been going to Dustin's boot camps for six months. I can do at least 20 push-ups with no problem now, whereas before I had to do them on my knees. I started with 15-pound weights and I am up to 20-pounders—sometimes even 25 pounds, depending on the exercise. And I just feel stronger. I can see toning in my arms and my abs. My legs aren't quite where I want them to be, but that's a work in progress.

"I'm more confident now. I've gone back to school for a further nursing degree. I have no problem wearing skirts and dresses and shorts outside because I am more toned. And emotionally, it's boosted my ego and made me happier. I'm a little more tired in the evenings because of those early-morning workouts, but I'm happier overall!"

Jenny's current goals: "I'd like to lose 10 more pounds and get into a size 10. And I want to continue working out three to five days per week even though I'm starting school."

Jenny's advice to you: "Just don't give up. There is always a way. You can't make any more excuses; you just have to get out and do it. Start slow if you have to. It doesn't happen overnight. But as long as you can get over that hump, it works."

Read more of Jenny's story at *fitmomsforlife.com/jenny.*

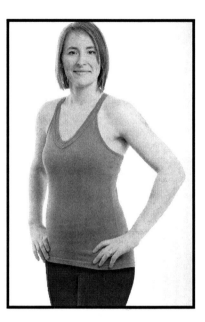

Jenny, 30, mother of three. 5'8", 160 pounds. Jenny went from a size 16 to a size 12 in six months of coming to my boot camps.

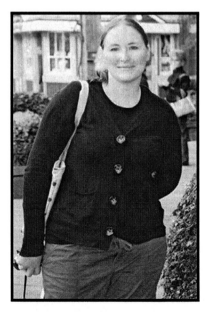

Fit Moms for Life Transformation

Patty

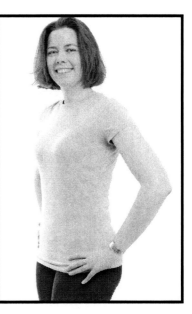

Patty was one of my original boot campers and has been coming for two and a half years. She's made an amazing physical transformation, going from a size 12 to a size 4.

Patty's story: "I was an avid swimmer from about six months old all the way through college. I avoided that dreaded 'freshman 15' because I was swimming all through college and stayed in great shape. But then I put on what I call the post-college 40, which is actually worse than the freshman 15. I really hadn't changed my eating habits from what they were when I was exercising all the time.

"I thought I was done with early-morning workouts when I stopped swimming, but my sister-in-law convinced me to come to boot camp with her when they were first starting up, in May 2008. I really went as a way to support my sister-in-law and help her get in shape. But a couple of months in, I started to feel stronger and lose some weight, and that's when I started to think it was a good way for me to get back into shape and to get back into some of the clothes I hadn't been able to wear since college.

"I could barely do two regular push-ups when I started. And after a couple months, I could do 10. Now I can do 50, 60 push-ups at a time. I've had to bust out the push-ups a couple of times in public because my friends are always bragging to other people that I can do them one-legged."

Patty's advice to you: "Don't gauge how much success you are or are not having by what other people are doing. You know, I lost 40 pounds. I went down four pants sizes. But I did that over almost two years. It was not a quick transition. Personally, I think slow is better, because it's a lot more maintainable. I developed habits that I can actually sustain now for the rest of my life."

Read more of Patty's story at *fitmomsforlife.com/pattyh.*

Patty, 28.
5'4", 125 pounds.
Patty lost 40 pounds and regained the athleticism she'd been missing since her competitive swimming days.

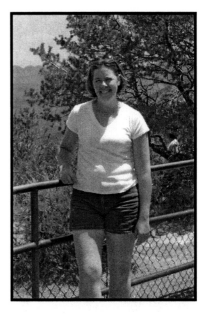

NUTRITION: EATING TO BE FIT FOR LIFE

"I was really amazed at how uninformed—and misinformed—I was about nutrition." – Mary

"You have to reevaluate what you are eating and think about food as fuel. What is the highest-quality fuel you can give your body?" – Crystal

"So many people go on a diet, as opposed to really changing the way that they eat. For me it had to be a journey, and if it weren't for the journey I don't think I would be where I am now." – Liz

Nutrition plays a huge role in your health and wellness, especially when it comes to losing weight and maintaining a healthy weight. A lot of people believe they can eat whatever they want if they're exercising enough. Unfortunately, that's not the case. This may sound odd coming from a personal trainer, but if I had to pick one or the other, I would tell you to eat well and not exercise. There are a lot of people in the world who maintain a healthy body weight by doing minimal exercise, such as walking daily, because they pay close attention to what they eat. Of course, I'd prefer that you do both! When you combine healthy eating with the right kind of exercise, you'll see amazing results.

I like to think of food as fuel. Your body is a machine that needs good-quality fuel to run optimally. You also need different types of fuel depending on what you are asking your body to do at different times of the day.

I don't have any pets, but I am amazed when I'm at a house where the owner freaks out if I try to feed the dog some table scraps or a treat because it isn't the healthiest food for the animal. Of course, this person and their family are usually eating food they know isn't the healthiest for human beings. I want to say, "Are you serious? Did you just demonstrate to me that you're more concerned about feeding your pet the proper nutrients than yourself and your family?" Unfortunately, this is the fact in many cases!

As you become more educated about nutrition, you become more critical of what you're putting in your body and when. That's not to say that you shouldn't enjoy food and take pleasure in what you're eating or that you can never have a treat. You need balance in what you eat. If you eat well most of the time, you will see a difference in how you feel and look. Healthy food can also taste great! But your focus needs to be on providing your body the energy it needs to do what you want to do.

In this section, I'll teach you the basic essential facts about nutrition, introduce you to my nutrition philosophy and rules for eating, provide a list of healthy foods to eat, and share some tips for making my eating plan work for you. Nutritional consultant Tracie Hittman Fountain, M.S., has created a set of meal and snack ideas and recipes that provide the right balance of protein, carbohydrates, and fat, including some gluten-free and dairy-free options. You'll find the meal ideas and recipes in Chapter 5 and snack ideas in Chapter 6.

Food as Fuel

Nutrition 101

Most people have heard of the three macronutrients: carbohydrates (or carbs), fats, and proteins. Most of my recommendations for what to eat are based on what percentage of your calories should come from each of these three macronutrient groups.

Carbohydrates provide your energy. One gram of carbohydrate equals 4 calories. More often than not, those calories go right into sustaining energy and keeping your body moving. But if you've already eaten enough and you don't need that energy, it's going to turn into fat. Carbohydrates have gotten a bad reputation recently, but your body needs them to function. By paying attention to the type and amount of carbohydrates you consume, when you consume them, and what else you're eating with them, you'll be able to keep your energy level consistent and your body from storing excess carbs as body fat.

The **fat** you consume is very important. Fat is very calorie-dense—it contains 9 calories per gram, so it's more than twice as calorie-dense as carbs and protein. People think that when you consume fat you're going to get fat, but fats are actually very important to a healthy diet. Fat is necessary for your hormones to work as they should, and low-fat diets can mess up your hormones pretty badly. Fat affects levels of estrogen, testosterone, cortisol, and the thyroid hormones. Fat also makes you feel full. I believe in a moderate-fat diet, which may be higher in fat than what some people would consider normal or healthy, as long as the fat is coming from healthy, natural sources.

The third macronutrient is **protein**. Like carbohydrates, protein contains 4 calories per gram. Protein is made up of different combinations of 20 amino acids that are basically the building blocks of your muscle. Your body uses protein to repair and build muscle after a strength training workout. Eating protein also increases your satiety, making you feel fuller. Protein also takes a lot of energy to break down. I recommend eating a lot of it to help you build muscle, feel full, and raise your metabolism.

In general, I recommend eating a balanced diet of carbs, fat, and protein. That means getting 30 to 40 percent of your calories from each macronutrient each day. You want roughly equal numbers of grams of protein and carbs (4 calories per gram), and a little less than half that many grams of fats (9 calories per gram). Some people do better with a higher-fat diet, some people do better with a higher-carb diet, and some do better with a higher-protein diet. You can play around with it to see what works best for you, but the 30-40 percent range for all three is a good place to start. If you follow the balanced diet for a month and you aren't seeing the results you want, you might start experimenting. Maybe reduce the carbs to 20 percent or increase them to 50 percent, or bump your protein up to 40 percent and just see how you feel and how your body responds. Don't make changes too frequently— give any plan a month before you decide whether it's right for you.

> " I had no idea how I should be eating. When I would try to diet, I would just count calories. Of course, now I know that doesn't work if you just eat 1,000 calories of carbs in a day. So that was a big eye-opener for me. Once I started learning about nutrition from Dustin, I started to eat a lot more protein, which kept me full."
>
> – Tiffany

Your body burns calories three ways, and this constitutes your metabolism. The biggest contributor to your caloric consumption is your basal metabolic rate, or BMR, which accounts for 60 percent of your metabolism. That is the energy your body needs to survive, or the calories you would use even if you slept all day. Your BMR decreases as you get older. It can also decrease if you eat a very low-calorie diet, as your body tries to conserve energy. You can increase your BMR through exercise and by building muscle, which takes more calories to maintain.

The next component of metabolism is activity, which includes everything you do besides sleeping: exercising, working, walking, driving, etc. This adds up to about 20 to 30 percent of the average person's energy consumption. (If you're very active—like training for an Ironman race or something similar—you might use as much as 60 to 70 percent of your calories on activity. If you lead a very sedentary lifestyle, this might drop as low as 15 percent.)

Finally, your body also uses calories to break down food in your body, in a process called thermogenesis. Thermogenesis only accounts for about 10 percent of your total metabolism. Protein requires more calories to break down than carbs and fats, so by eating a high-protein diet, you can increase the calories your body burns in thermogenesis.[1]

---

1 Halton, T.L., and F.B. Hu. "The Effects of High Protein Diets on Thermogenesis, Satiety and Weight Loss: A Critical Review." Journal of the American College of Nutrition 23.5 (2004): 373-85.

The last things I want to explain about nutrition are blood sugar levels and the glycemic index. Each time you eat, as the food (or liquid) is digested in your stomach, it gets broken down and absorbed into your bloodstream. When carbohydrates hit your bloodstream—especially simple carbs like sugar, fruits and fruit juices, processed grains, and white flour—your blood sugar level rises and insulin is released to bring it back down. Insulin pulls sugar into your liver and your muscles first, because both of those areas need sugar. But if you're consuming more sugar and simple carbs than your liver and muscles need, they will be stored as fat instead.

Obviously, that's not what we want to happen. But that's not the only problem with this scenario. When your blood contains high levels of glucose (sugar) and the insulin comes out in full force, your blood sugar levels drop quickly and you crash. That's when your mood drops, your energy drops, and you have a harder time thinking clearly. You become hungry again, and your body wants you to eat again to get your blood sugar levels back up. Repeating this cycle over and over again can also lead to insulin resistance, diabetes, and other health problems. You're much better off if you can keep your blood sugar levels steady throughout the day and avoid those highs and crashes.

> *I had bad habits, and I didn't even know it. I thought I was doing myself a favor when in the middle of the day I'd eat an orange or an apple. But now I know you have to ground that with a protein, so you don't spike your blood sugar. I was just coming from a point of knowing nothing about what I should've been eating."*
>
> – Trish

Different foods have different effects on your blood sugar levels. The glycemic index indicates how much your blood sugar levels increase when you eat a particular food item. Basically, the more glucose in the food, the higher your blood sugar will go, and the higher the glycemic index rating will be. There is a lot of variation even among similar types of foods. For example: bananas, oranges, and grapes have relatively high glycemic index ratings, whereas berries, apples, and pears are lower. The lower-glycemic-index foods usually have more fiber in them, which helps temper the effect on your blood sugar level. Most vegetables have a lower glycemic index than most fruits. Most of the dark leafy greens, sweet potatoes, and other vegetables with rich color are lower-glycemic and lower-carb in general. Understanding the glycemic index can help you make better choices and put together meals that will help keep your blood sugar levels steady. The lower the glycemic number, the better. Visit *glycemicindex.com* for GIs of common foods.

My Nutrition Philosophy: The Low-Crap Diet

My approach to nutrition is basically that people should be eating as all-natural as possible and be aware of what they're eating. I don't recommend a low-fat diet or a low-protein diet or a low-carb diet—but I do like to say we should all be eating a low-crap diet. That means eating food that is as natural and as whole as possible, going back to the basics, and eating the way God intended us to eat.

Being aware of what you're eating isn't just about reading ingredient labels, though that's a big part of it. It is also about paying attention to portion sizes, keeping a food journal, and noticing when something other than hunger is driving you to eat—in other words, eating consciously. You may have read or heard some of this before, but I'm going to provide a structure that will help you actually put that knowledge to use.

Rules to Eat By

Here are the 16 rules that I believe are the cornerstone of what you should be doing. If you do these things most of the time, you're going to get great results, you're going to feel better, and you're going to have more energy! If you're not ready to change everything at once, that's fine. Just pick a few rules to start following this month, add a few more next month, and so on.

Rules to Eat By

1. Don't eat carbs alone.
2. If you can't pronounce the ingredients, don't eat it.
3. If your great-grandma didn't eat it, don't eat it.
4. Eat breakfast.
5. Eat four to six small meals per day.
6. Keep your portion size under control.
7. Drink three to four quarts of water each day.
8. Don't drink calories (juice, soda, alcohol).
9. Avoid fake sugars.
10. Eat enough protein.
11. Don't eat grains after 4 p.m.
12. Be careful what you eat in the evening.
13. Give yourself two to three cheat meals per week.
14. Be prepared.
15. Eat grass-fed meat and free-range poultry.
16. Buy organic when possible and practical.

---

1. Don't eat carbs alone. The foods we think of as being made up mostly of carbs—like bread, grains, and some fruits—contain large amounts of sugar, which will cause your blood sugar levels to rise very quickly. As I described above, not only is your body likely to store that sugar as fat, but you're also going to crash after a little while. And then it becomes a vicious cycle, because what are you going to reach for when you're grumpy, low on energy, and not thinking clearly? More carbs! And here we go again. This may sound familiar to you—and everyone else who heads to the office vending machines or sneaks a sugary treat while her kids are napping in the mid-afternoon.

The key to having the most energy throughout the day is to keep your blood sugar levels as consistent as possible. When your blood sugar levels look like a roller coaster, going up and down throughout the day, you're on that ride emotionally and physically. An all-day, everyday roller coaster isn't any fun, and it's also not good for maintaining a healthy weight. So what we need to do is combine those carbs with a protein or a fat. (Use the list of healthy carbs, fats, and proteins on page 71, and always be sure to combine something from the carbs list with something from the fats or proteins list every time you eat.)

Fats and proteins stay in your stomach longer and take much longer for your body to absorb, and don't affect your blood sugar as drastically as carbs. Let's say you eat a bagel and a banana for breakfast. Your body has to deal with a lot of carbs all at once, with very little protein or fat to slow down the absorption. But if you have a couple of eggs and a banana, the protein and fat in the eggs make it take much longer for all that sugar to get released into the body, meaning you're not going to experience an extreme blood sugar rush and subsequent crash. You're going to feel fuller longer, too.

I've heard from people who have made this change without altering anything else about how they eat, and they report a decent amount of weight loss relatively rapidly. It can make a huge difference, because you're not storing that sugar as fat, and you're not experiencing the roller coaster that leads to more poor food choices.

I should mention that there's a little bit of controversy around this rule. Some people say it's okay to eat fruit alone, since it doesn't contain processed sugars and has more fiber. To me, regardless of what type of carb it is, it's going to raise your blood sugar levels and set the same process in motion. Have a piece of fruit with a cheese stick or a small handful of nuts and see how you feel.

2. If you can't pronounce the ingredients, don't eat it. This rule and the next one are recommended by Michael Pollan in his book *Food Rules: An Eater's Manual*. They are really key to a low-crap diet. First of all, eat things you can pronounce. Read the ingredient list on a product. If it contains ingredients you can't pronounce or understand, you probably shouldn't be eating it. Most of those ingredients are chemicals or preservatives put in the food to increase its shelf life. They're not food. You want to focus on whole foods and products that are made from whole foods.

> *If you don't recognize the ingredients, do you really want to be eating it?"*
> – Tina

3. If your great-grandma didn't eat it, don't eat it. Michael Pollan also talks about eating things your grandma would recognize. I'd go so far as to suggest your great-grandma, because depending on your age, your grandma might have gotten most of her food out of boxes and cans. Of course, this goes with the previous rule. Eighty or 90 years ago, your great-grandma couldn't conceive of most of the ingredients in today's commercially produced yogurt, for example, or other highly processed foods. Sticking with food that's been around for a long time will basically keep you away from those highly processed foods, and you're going to be a lot better off for it. (By the way, with these two rules, I don't mean to say you shouldn't try anything new or enjoy foods from other cultures just because you don't recognize it. Definitely try new things and new flavors—just stick to those that are made from whole foods and aren't overly processed!)

4. Eat breakfast. You've probably been hearing this one since elementary school, so I'm not going to beat a dead horse, but it is so important to eat breakfast. It really has been shown to be the most important meal of the day. This is because you're breaking a fast: Your blood sugar levels are definitely low after eight to 12 hours without food, so you need to get something in your body to bring them up soon after you rise. Eating breakfast also decreases the likelihood that you will overeat later in the day. You've probably tried this—you skip breakfast, but by noon you're really hungry, so you eat a big meal for lunch, and by the time you get to dinner, you're really, really hungry because you've gone all day with just one meal. So you end up eating a huge meal at night, not long before you go to sleep, when you won't be burning those calories. That's not the best way to go about it.

You also have to remember Rule 1 with this: When you eat breakfast, don't eat carbs alone. A good breakfast might be two whole eggs with a piece of sprouted whole-grain toast and a quarter to half of an avocado. The eggs provide protein and a little bit of fat. The toast provides carbs—and bread made from sprouted grains has less of an effect on your blood sugar than processed grains. The avocado provides additional healthy fats. This breakfast is going to keep your blood sugar levels fairly steady without ever getting super-high. It's going to take a long time for all that to break down in your body. You're going to have sustained energy for many hours with a breakfast like that.

5. Eat four to six small meals per day. Eating small meals frequently is another strategy for maintaining your blood sugar levels. You're not overloading your body with a huge meal two or three times a day and then getting really hungry in between. You're eating every three to four hours and avoiding those big swings in blood sugar levels. It helps me to know I'm always going to have another meal in about three hours, so I don't feel like I have to stuff my face. Even if I don't feel super-full from what I just ate, that's okay, because within three hours I'll get some more food.

6. Keep your portion size under control. This is closely related to Rule 5—if you're going to eat frequently throughout the day, you really can't eat huge portions. I talk to a lot of people who say, "I think I eat pretty healthy; I just eat too much of it." That can definitely be the case. One of my clients had lost 20 pounds under my coaching, but then had plateaued. She was getting frustrated because she was doing all the right things exercise-wise. And the foods she was eating were healthy. I had her do a food journal and weigh her food and calculate her calories. Well, there was a salad she loved to make for lunch. It was a really hearty one, with nuts on it and all kinds of good things. Once she weighed each thing she was putting on it, she figured out she was eating an 800-calorie salad for lunch every day. She usually had a couple other healthy things on the side, so she was typically consuming 1,000 calories just from lunch. Yes, she was eating the healthy, whole foods I recommend—but if you're trying to eat 1,500 or 1,800 calories a day, you can't really afford to use half or more of them on one salad!

We have a pretty skewed sense of portion size in our culture right now. Some restaurants include five servings of pasta in the big bowl they sell as a single meal! It's just ridiculous. Dinner plates are bigger now. Everything is "super-sized." To get your sense of portion size back on track, I'd recommend a couple of things. First, get your

> *It's about making better choices and eating small quantities. I don't need a huge amount of food to be satisfied."*
> – Sandra

food scale out and weigh things. That's going to be your best bet. If you don't have a scale or you don't have it with you, you can go by the following visual guidelines: A portion size of a vegetable or fruit is roughly the size of your fist. That's about a cup for most vegetables. The same rule goes for carbs like bread, pasta, rice, or potatoes—a portion is about the size of your fist. For meat, poultry, or fish, a serving is about the size of a deck of playing cards or the palm of your hand. A portion of fat is about the size of your pinky or somewhere between a teaspoon and a tablespoon. For most of your meals, you want to have about one portion of protein, one portion of carbs, one to two portions of vegetables, and a portion of fat.

7. Drink three to four quarts of water each day. Here's another one you've probably heard before. There is definitely conflicting research out there about how much water we need for optimal

health, and newer studies say we don't need as much as was recommended before. But I still drink three to four quarts of water each day and tell my clients to do the same. (You can also take half of your weight and aim to drink that many ounces of water each day.) Maybe it's a little bit old-school, but I haven't seen any negative side effects besides having to go to the bathroom a lot. It'll keep you hydrated, of course, but I think it cuts down on cravings too, and helps you feel fuller. I just feel better and cleaner when I drink enough water.

> *Water is so much easier to grab than a can of soda. Plus, you save tons of money by not drinking it. I always keep pitchers of water in the refrigerator. So whenever somebody is thirsty, they pour it in a glass, refill it, so easy, so nice. Makes you feel clean."*
> – Jody

The best way to do it is to use a quart water bottle, fill it up in the morning, and just keep drinking and refilling it throughout your day. Always keep it in front of you. If it's not around, you're not thinking about it, and you won't think to drink water until you feel really thirsty; by that time your body is becoming dehydrated. If you get bored from drinking plain water, there are some ways to make it a little bit more exciting. You can put some lemon or cucumber slices in it. You can make green tea or other varieties of tea that don't include any additives. Just keep the water going throughout the day. You might have to work up to drinking three to four quarts per day, so just slowly increase your water each day until you hit that amount.

8. Don't drink calories (juice, soda, alcohol). The problem with drinking calories is that they send sugar into your bloodstream and don't make your body feel full. Many people think juice is healthy because it's made from fruit. (By the way, check the label of the juice you buy and see whether it is 100 percent fruit juice or if it contains added sugar and preservatives!) I'm not saying it's bad for you in moderation, but I've met people who were drinking almost a gallon of orange juice a day and not understanding why they couldn't lose weight. Now, if you're juicing fresh fruits, and especially if you're adding in vegetables, it's a little bit different; but in general, when you drink juice, you're not getting the fiber and some of the nutrients that are in the peel. I'd always recommend a piece of whole fruit rather than a glass of juice.

> I don't always get as much water in as I should, but I can tell the difference when I do. I'm not hungry at all."
>
> – Amber

Then we have soda—or pop, as I like to call it, because I'm from Minnesota. Soda is one of America's favorite sources of empty calories. Everyone knows soda isn't good, because of its high sugar content and all the chemicals used to make it. (A lot of people still believe diet soda is good for them. We're going to talk about fake sugars in the next rule. For now, let's just say that if you're going to drink a soda every once in a while, I'd rather see you drink the regular stuff and avoid the fake sugars in diet soda.)

The other main liquid source of empty calories is alcohol. Besides being a sugar with little nutrient value, alcohol has the added bonus of lowering your inhibitions, which leads a lot of people to make poor food choices once they've been drinking. I know there are a lot of studies out there that say a glass of wine in the evening is good for the heart or for your cholesterol. I'm not denying that. I think a couple of drinks a week is fine, and some people can handle that better than others. Some people report that when they stop drinking altogether, they see a fair amount of weight loss. Obviously, when people are overdrinking, we all know that's not healthy for you. You're damaging your liver and you're also making bad eating choices, generally when you're drinking a lot. The phrase "beer belly" exists for a reason. Studies show that the people who drink the most—especially those who drink a lot of beer—do get that fat accumulation around their gut. It's a lot harder to have a lean, flat stomach if you're drinking a lot of alcohol.

Now, if you're going to drink juice, soda, or alcohol occasionally, the most important thing is to go back to Rule 1. You need to combine it with a protein or a fat to decrease the chance of all that sugar getting stored as body fat right away. With juice and soda, I'd also say your best bet is to have those sugary drinks right before or after working out, so that your muscles absorb the sugar quickly.

By the way, I get a lot of questions about kids and juice. If you're going to get juice for your kids, be sure to buy 100 percent real fruit juice. Some moms dilute juice with water, and their kids never know the difference. Other than that, the same rules apply. Kids are just like adults in the sense that if you give them a lot of sugar, they're going to get a sugar high and then they're going to crash. So you want to combine any juice they drink with a fat or protein.

9. Avoid fake sugars. As I mentioned above, I'm not a fan of artificial sweeteners or fake sugars. They come in a lot of different forms—aspartame and sucralose are the most common ones you'll find in diet sodas and many "sugar-free" or "no sugar added" products, including a lot of yogurts and many protein powders. The research out there is inconclusive as to whether fake sugars cause diseases like cancer and Alzheimer's. But the way I see it, all those chemicals are foreign to your body. They are toxic things your body doesn't know what to do with. I don't even touch them for that reason alone.

But there is also a lot of evidence to suggest that consuming fake sugars is counterproductive from a weight-loss perspective. Research on rats has shown that consuming fake sugars increases calorie consumption, weight gain, and body fat. Rats that were fed fake sugars consumed more calories later on than rats that were not.[2] We also know from human studies that people with high levels of fake sugar in their diets are more likely to be overweight.[3] Now, there could be a lot of psychological and behavioral reasons for that. Many times, people who eat a lot of "diet" food believe they're making up

> *You have to give up the drinks with fake sugar, even though they're zero calories and you think they're not making any difference. I was a Diet Pepsi and Crystal Light addict. When I gave those up, I noticed a huge difference. That's when the weight really started to come off."*
>
> – Donna

for eating other bad food—so they had the diet soda and low-calorie yogurt in the afternoon and then feel justified eating pizza for dinner. But as the research with the rats shows, there may be some physiological things going on as well that make fake sugars ineffective as a weight-loss tool. So try to get rid of them. Stevia would be a good calorie-free natural sweetener choice.

10. Eat enough protein. We've already talked about how protein helps you feel fuller for longer and how it burns more calories than other types of food. There are many different viewpoints on how much protein you need. If you talk to the majority of mainstream nutritionists or you look at the government's nutritional guidelines, the advice is to eat a very grain-based diet that is not particularly high in protein. I'm not going to get into the politics I believe are behind those

2 Swithers, S.E., C.R. Baker, and T.L. Davidson. "General and Persistent Effects of High-Intensity Sweeteners on Body Weight Gain and Caloric Compensation in Rats." Behavioral Neuroscience 123.4 (2009): 772-80.

3 Lutsey, P.L., L.M. Steffen, and J. Stevens. "Dietary Intake and the Development of the Metabolic Syndrome: The Atherosclerosis Risk in Communities Study." Circulation 117 (2008): 754-61.

recommendations; I'll just say that research has shown that higher amounts of protein are linked to lower body fat. So I promote a high-protein diet. I tell people to try to get 1 gram of protein per pound of their ideal body weight each day. If your ideal weight would be 150 pounds, try to get about 150 grams of protein. If you break that down into your four to six meals, you want to average about 30 grams of protein each time you eat. I've worked with nutritionists who tell me their clients often struggle to get 30, 40, or 50 grams of protein a day. You're not going to feel full from that. You're certainly not going to be able to build muscle from it. Your body's going to be atrophying.

11. Don't eat grains after 4 p.m. As a general rule, I avoid grains and starchy carbs in the evening. This means no bread, pasta, or rice with dinner and no sweets after dinner. I don't even like to eat fruit after 4 p.m., because my body doesn't need that type of fuel for the level of activity I engage in most evenings. This rule doesn't apply if you're working out later in the evening, because you definitely want to have some simple carbs as an energy source for your workout. But if you're not working out and you're not very active after you come home from work or pick up the kids from all their activities, watch your carbs closely. That's when you run the risk of storing carbs as fat because you aren't using your muscles and your body isn't looking for that fast energy. Your dinners should really be made up of lean protein and a little bit of fat, and then a lot of non-starchy vegetables, like asparagus, broccoli, spinach, and hearty lettuces. Those foods have a lot of nutrients without a lot of calories, and they're going to have very low carbs in them, too. This gets us back to the glycemic index. Especially later in the day, you want to choose carbs that have a lower glycemic index, more fiber, and fewer carbs. I'm not opposed to people eating regular potatoes, but sweet potatoes or yams are a much better option, especially in the evening. Calorie-wise they're about the same, but the latter have higher fiber and more nutrients.

> *Eat more protein than you are probably currently eating. I try to aim for 20 grams of protein per meal or snack. When you're getting that much protein, you feel more full."*
>
> – Kelly

12. Be careful what you eat in the evening. Some experts discourage eating later at night or after supper. I wouldn't say you shouldn't eat after supper if you like to stay up late, but what you're eating after supper matters. It should be a balanced snack or small meal just like you eat the rest of the day. A lot of people eat sugar or processed fats, cookies, chips, ice cream, and that sort of thing as they're sitting in front of the TV at night. Some people link this to not getting enough protein early in the day. Try increasing your protein at breakfast and see if those late-night cravings go away. Think about what type of fuel your body needs at the end of the day. One great food for later in the evening is cottage cheese. Cottage cheese does have some natural carbs from lactose, but it has high levels of casein protein, which breaks down really slowly in your body. So it's one of the best things to eat before you go to sleep, because those proteins will circulate through your bloodstream throughout the night, for four to six hours. (In comparison, whey protein will break down within about an hour.) You could eat some turkey or any sort of meat, or some raw almonds. I'd say you want to have between 100 and 200 calories. That should feed you through the night, and you should wake up in the morning feeling hungry but not ravenous.

13. Give yourself two to three cheat meals per week. There are a lot of different reasons for giving yourself some cheat meals every week, both psychological and physiological. First, if I said you could never eat dessert again, or french fries, or whatever food it is that you really enjoy, you would probably feel really deprived, and you'd rebel and binge at some point. You might not even try the program in the first place. So you have to allow yourself to eat something that's less virtuous every once in a while.

Also, if you're on a lower-calorie diet, at some point your body will start to conserve energy. That's not a good thing, because it's going to start to store fat. So what we need to do is shock the system every once in a while and let your body know you're not in a famine—you've just chosen not to eat as much. So about once a week we bump those calories up for a few meals, and your body kind of resets itself and realizes it's not starving, and will continue burning fat at a higher level.

Knowing it's okay to cheat occasionally is also what makes my program realistic for your life. There are holidays, birthdays, and special events when you want to be able to eat special foods without feeling like you're breaking the rules or derailing your diet. How many times have you said you can't start your diet until after the holidays? How many times have you thrown all your good habits out the window because of a meal or a day when you didn't eat well? You won't have that excuse with this plan. Just count it as your cheat meal or cheat day and get back with the program the next day!

There's one other thing about cheat days. Let's say you totally pig out for one day and enjoy everything you feel you're missing out on the rest of the time. I guarantee that if you're eating well the rest of the week, you're going to feel awful after that binge. You're going to be bloated. You're going to have gas. You're probably going to have low energy. You're going to feel stuffed. It helps you realize how much better you feel when you eat well. A lot of people actually can't wait to get back on the wagon after their cheat day!

> " *Don't deprive yourself. If you want to have a treat once in a while—not every day, not three times a day, but once in a while—that's okay. You will make yourself crazy if you try to stick to a perfect diet all the time."*
> – Kelly

In terms of how to do your cheat meals, I recommend ignoring the rules for two to three meals per week and trying to keep those all on the same day. Another way to think about it is to try to maintain 85 percent compliance to my rules each week. That gives you wiggle room to eat some of your favorite foods or celebrate a special event without going overboard. Around the holidays or during other busy times, my recommendation is to eat 100 percent clean whenever you're at home or preparing your own food, saving all your cheating for parties and events.

Be careful not to give yourself the whole weekend "off." I've seen a lot of clients who lose one to two pounds between Monday and Friday and then gain it all back on the weekend. So they're putting in all that hard work during the week to lose the same two pounds over and over! (If you do this but only check your weight once a week or less, it looks like your weight is just staying constant.) My friend and fat loss expert Joel Marion became famous for his *Cheat Your Way Thin* Program, where he shows you what cheat foods you can eat and still lose fat. You can pick up his program up at *cheatyourwaythin.com*.

14. Be prepared. It's not hard to eat the way I'm recommending, but it does take preparation. You aren't going to find many acceptable foods in a vending machine or at a convenience store. I think the most important tip of all is knowing what your day is going to be like and preparing either the night before or on the weekend. Preparing means planning what you will eat for each meal, as well as spending the time shopping and preparing food so that you can follow through with that plan.

I encourage you to take some time on Sunday to look at your week and plan your meals—not just your dinners, but also what you need to have on hand for all your other meals. Think about how you will get your protein in for each meal and what vegetables you will be eating. Then go buy a lot of your ingredients and the foods you're going to need for the week or the next few days. I recommend you do some precooking. Cook as much as you can in one day, making big batches and putting things in the fridge and freezer for later in the week. Then you won't give in to temptation to eat unhealthily, because everything is ready to go. Stash some raw almonds in your purse or your car so that you're never caught off guard. I'll talk about other ways to be prepared in the next chapter.

> " Every weekend I make a meal plan for the week and make the grocery list with that, because your days get busier as the week goes on, and then you just rush and grab something quick. If you have a plan and all the ingredients you need, it's much simpler to make that healthy choice."
>
> – Karen E.

15. Eat grass-fed meat and free-range poultry. I've focused on this more in the past year. I love meat, and I don't think I'll ever become a vegetarian. But now I focus on eating grass-fed beef and free-range or pastured chicken and eggs. Some people have philosophical and ethical reasons for doing this, but it also makes a big difference for your health. The fatty acid profile in a grass-fed cow is completely different from in a grain-fed cow. It's almost like salmon from the ocean, in terms of the omega-3 and omega-6 fatty acids you're getting. My good friend Mike Geary, author of the ebook *Truth About Six Pack Abs* (*truthaboutabs.com*), goes in depth on the benefits of grass-fed meat compared to corn- and soybean-fed. The same thing is true with egg yolks. In an egg from a chicken that has roamed around eating grass and bugs, the yolk has a very healthy fatty acid profile, including more omega-3s and less cholesterol than you get from conventional eggs. Eggs from pastured chickens are also filled with many more vitamins and nutrients than conventional eggs. Conventional meat and poultry are raised on corn and soybeans now, which is not what those animals were meant to eat; I believe that's detrimental to their health and metabolism as well as to ours. (The documentary *Food, Inc.* describes all of this and makes these points really well.)

So my advice is to buy local, like at a farmer's market or right from a farm, where you can ask the farmer how the meat, poultry, or eggs are produced. That's the ideal. (The labels "free range" and "cage-free" on chicken and eggs just mean the chickens have access to the outdoors. They do not say anything about how they were fed or whether they actually spent any time outside. Ask the farmer whether his or her chickens are pastured, or what they eat.) I know in some places this can be hard to do. If you can't buy these foods locally, find online sources. Yes, it's more expensive, but I think it's worth it for the difference it will make in your health. You'll get more nutritional bang for your buck. And you can make it less expensive if you're able to buy it in bulk. For example, you can buy a full butchered beef and split it up with family or friends, or buy a quarter of one and put it all in the freezer. You can buy poultry in bulk, too. When you do that, it really becomes almost comparable, price-wise, to the stuff you buy in the stores.

16. Buy organic when possible and practical. There are a lot of different opinions about how important it is to buy organic, how bad pesticides are for us, and how much pesticide residues there are in our food. I take a middle road. I go by the "Dirty Dozen" and "Clean 15" lists from the Environmental Working Group (see the 2011 lists on page 68), which list the fruits and vegetables grown with the highest and lowest levels of pesticides in conventional farming. The Dirty Dozen are the ones I buy organic. The Clean 15 are the ones I don't worry about as much. My advice is to spend your money first on the higher-quality, grass-fed, and free-range meat and poultry as I described in Rule 15, and then add organic fruits and vegetables if you can afford it, starting with the ones at the top of the Dirty Dozen list. Make sure to compare prices of organic and conventional produce when you shop. Often, organic food on sale is cheaper than its conventional counterparts. In addition, seasonal produce is usually the cheaper and more nutritious way to go.

If you really can't afford to buy organic foods, that's fine. Just focus on getting fresher, less processed food. Use a vegetable wash to clean non-organic fruits and veggies. Try to eat more items from the Clean 15 list and fewer from the Dirty Dozen to reduce your pesticide exposure. It's definitely a continuum, and I'm not saying you have to be perfect. There's really no end to the number of pesticides and chemicals we encounter every day in our modern lives. So you have to make the changes you can and be practical about it. You've got to do what is good and right for your family.

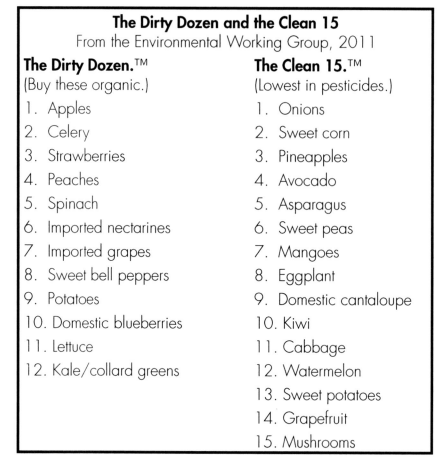

The Dirty Dozen and the Clean 15
From the Environmental Working Group, 2011

The Dirty Dozen.™
(Buy these organic.)

1. Apples
2. Celery
3. Strawberries
4. Peaches
5. Spinach
6. Imported nectarines
7. Imported grapes
8. Sweet bell peppers
9. Potatoes
10. Domestic blueberries
11. Lettuce
12. Kale/collard greens

The Clean 15.™
(Lowest in pesticides.)

1. Onions
2. Sweet corn
3. Pineapples
4. Avocado
5. Asparagus
6. Sweet peas
7. Mangoes
8. Eggplant
9. Domestic cantaloupe
10. Kiwi
11. Cabbage
12. Watermelon
13. Sweet potatoes
14. Grapefruit
15. Mushrooms

Foods to Avoid

There are really only a few foods I would say you should never eat or eat as little of as possible. First, limit your consumption of foods that contain trans fats. Those are the highly processed fats that have received a lot of attention in the news lately. A lot of fried foods, doughnuts, and other baked goods with a long shelf life have trans fats in them—indicated by the words "partially hydrogenated" oils in the ingredient list. Unfortunately, trans fat substitutes used in manufactured baked goods may have negative health effects similar to those of trans fats,[4] so it's probably best to steer clear of those products in general.

Soy is another ingredient I encourage everyone to research and eat with caution. This book is not about soy, so I'll just say you should read up on it. It's very controversial. But it is pretty clear that our society has consumed huge amounts of soy in the last 20 to 30 years. It is very processed soy, and we get it in everything, from the meats we eat to breads and processed foods. That's on top of

4 Vega-Lopez, Sonia, et al. "Palm and Partially Hydrogenated Soybean Oils Adversely Alter Lipoprotein Profiles Compared with Soybean and Canola Oils in Moderately Hyperlipidemic Subjects." The American Journal of Clinical Nutrition 84.1 (2006): 54-62.

the soy milk and Boca Burgers and tofu people eat in an attempt to be healthy. I believe we're seeing estrogenic changes in both women and men as a result. Increased levels of estrogen increase the level of fat in your body. I stay away from soy whenever I can, especially the more processed forms.

The other things I steer clear of are fake sugars and chemicals in general, as I mentioned above. Other than that, I don't consider any food off limits. Let's say you love ice cream. Who doesn't love ice cream on a hot summer day? Sure, it's not the best food for you, if you eat tons of it. But I see no problem with enjoying it in moderation, as long as you choose ice cream that has all-natural ingredients—you know, the ones your great-grandma would recognize—like Breyer's Natural or Häagen-Dazs.

Keep a Food Journal

One of the most powerful things you can do to help yourself become more aware of what you're eating is to keep a food journal. Among people trying to lose weight, studies have shown that those who consistently keep a food journal lose up to twice as much weight as those who don't.[5] This isn't anything new and groundbreaking, and you've probably heard it before. But you will get so much out of it if you just commit to doing it!

In Chapter 4, I explained how to keep your food journal and described some of the technology available to make it easier. The difference at this point in the program is that, rather than just trying to record what you're eating, you're now using your journal to help you eat better. The main benefit of keeping a food journal is that just by writing down everything you eat, you become more aware of how you're fueling your body. As my client Jenny said, "It gets you to really think before you eat something. If you see a piece of candy or a chocolate, you're more apt to say, 'Do I really need that now?'" It really helps cut down on mindless eating.

As I described in Chapter 4, a detailed food journal will also allow you to calculate how many calories you're eating in a day. It's also really useful when you can see the breakdown of carbs, fats, and proteins in your diet, so that you can aim for balance. Vanessa told me she thinks of her food journal like a checkbook she has to balance: "It keeps my portions in check, but I also like to look back on the day and say, 'Oh, I haven't eaten very many vegetables today,' or 'I really haven't eaten protein for a while.'"

A food journal is also a great way to provide yourself with some accountability, by showing it to someone else. Whether you're going to share it with a nutritionist, a personal trainer, or just a friend who might not even know that much about nutrition, just knowing that someone else is going to look at your food journal can help you make better choices. And the feedback you get from someone else looking at your journal might help you identify habits that aren't healthy or notice patterns in how you're eating and where your willpower is breaking down.

---

5 Hollis, J. "Weight Loss During the Intensive Intervention Phase of the Weight-Loss Maintenance Trial." American Journal of Preventive Medicine 35.2 (2008): 118-26.

I'd recommend you keep close track for about a week of following my program. (You can use the blank food journal on page 177 or download additional pages at *fitmomsforlife.com/foodjournal*.) That will give you a good sense of portion size and nutritional breakdowns. Then you may not need to continue keeping a detailed food journal, but every once in a while—especially if you start to feel yourself slip—go back to it and keep yourself on track that way.

My nutritional consultant, Tracie Hittman Fountain, also recommends keeping a "feelings journal." You can keep it separate from your food journal, but I like to consolidate them. Throughout the whole day, write down how you're feeling, your energy levels, your mood—maybe whether you're irritated, if you're tired, different things like that. If you do this long enough, you'll start to see patterns arise. You might realize you're having indigestion or feeling constipated when you eat gluten products or dairy, for example. Or you might notice that on the days you ate a well-balanced breakfast of carbs, fats and proteins, you felt great. Whereas the days you just ate cereal, a banana, and orange juice, you crashed later and couldn't concentrate. This will help you become really aware of your body and how it responds to certain foods.

A feelings journal also helps if you tend to be an emotional eater. A lot of women eat when they're stressed out, sad, or bored. So, if you write down what you're feeling or what happened before you went for the chips or the ice cream, you might find some patterns that are surprising. Writing it down might even help you catch yourself and realize you're not hungry and don't need to eat.

> " For me it's not that hard to eat healthy, but there are a lot of emotions that go with my body changing, how I feel when I exercise, and the struggles I have with my health problems. I use my food journal to write down not just what I'm eating and drinking, but also how I'm feeling as all of this is going on. I can look back at it and see that there were times when I felt really challenged, but that then I felt so much success afterward. That really helps."
>
> – Patrice

Eating Plan

Each time you eat, you should include foods from at least two of the macronutrient categories in the list of healthy carbs, fats, and proteins on page 71. Once you have the hang of it, you'll be creating your own meals and finding and adapting recipes that meet these standards. In the meantime, we wanted to give you a lot of examples to help you get started, Tracie Hittman Fountain has created lists of meals and snacks and is providing recipes for those that require preparation.

The idea is that each day you choose one breakfast option, one lunch option, and one dinner option from the meals listed on page 73 . You should also have one to three snacks, which are listed on page 86 in Chapter 6, for a total of four to six small meals per day. The meals include gluten-free options and dairy-free options because so many people have trouble processing one or both of those ingredients.

Healthy Carbs, Fats, and Proteins to Include in Your Eat...
(not an exhaustive list)

Carbs
Whole Grains
- Barley
- Brown rice
- Buckwheat
- Corn
- Millet
- Oats
- Quinoa
- Rye
- Spelt
- Whole wheat

Beans and Legumes
- Black beans
- Dried peas
- Garbanzo beans/chickpeas
- Kidney beans
- Lentils
- Lima beans
- Miso
- Navy beans
- Pinto beans

Fruits
- Apples
- Apricots
- Bananas
- Blueberries
- Cantaloupe
- Cranberries
- Figs
- Grapefruits
- Grapes
- Kiwifruits
- Lemons
- Limes
- Oranges
- Papayas
- Pears
- Pineapples
- Plums
- Prunes
- Raisins
- Raspberries
- Strawberries
- Watermelon

Natural Sweeteners
(use sparingly)
- Blackstrap molasses
- Cane juice
- Honey
- Maple syrup
- Stevia
- Xylitol

Vegetables (starchy)
- Carrots
- Green peas
- Potatoes
- Squash, winter
- Sweet potatoes
- Tomatoes
- Yams

Vegetables (non-starchy)
- Asparagus
- Avocado (healthy fat)
- Beets
- Bell peppers
- Broccoli
- Brussels sprouts
- Cabbage
- Cauliflower
- Celery
- Collard greens
- Cucumbers
- Eggplant
- Fennel
- Garlic
- Green beans
- Kale
- Leeks
- Mushrooms
- Mustard greens
- Olives
- Onions
- Parsley
- Romaine lettuce
- Sea vegetables
- Spinach
- Squash, summer
- Swiss chard
- Turnip greens

Fats
Nuts and See...
- Almonds
- Cashews
- Flaxseeds
- Peanuts
- Pistachios
- Pumpkin seeds
- Sesame seeds
- Sunflower seeds
- Walnuts

Oils
- Butter
- Coconut oil
- Olive oil, extra virgin

Protein
Poultry and Lean Meats
(grass-fed/pastured/organic)
- Beef, lean
- Calf's liver
- Chicken
- Lamb
- Turkey
- Venison

Fish and Seafood (wild-caught)
- Cod
- Halibut
- Salmon
- Scallops
- Shrimp
- Snapper
- Tilapia
- Tuna

Dairy
- Cheese
- Eggs
- Milk, 2% or full fat, cow's
- Milk, goat's
- Yogurt (plain)
- Greek yogurt (plain)
- Cottage cheese, 2% or full fat

Other
- Casein protein powder
- Hydrolyzed gelatin
- Whey protein powder

my clients have found that they feel better and lose weight quickly once they eliminate and/or dairy from their diets. You might want to give it a try for two or three weeks to see if makes a difference for you. (If you eliminate dairy from your diet long-term, be sure to replace it with other good sources of calcium.)

You might be surprised at a few of the items included in the list of healthy foods on page 71. Let me briefly discuss some of those foods and why they should be included in your healthy eating plan.

Butter. I believe all-natural fats are the best for you. I don't use products like margarine, made with chemical ingredients. I do use good old-fashioned butter, which has one ingredient—maybe two, if it's salted butter—and tastes great. If you can get organic butter from grass-fed cows, even better. Of course, many people are concerned about the cholesterol in butter. In the medical community, there is no real agreement about whether the cholesterol in your diet will increase your body's cholesterol level. I believe that it doesn't, but you may have to test that with a little caution if you have high cholesterol issues.

Coconut oil. Another fat I like to use, especially for cooking, is coconut oil. Coconut oil is making a comeback; it went out of fashion for a while because it is a saturated fat. But it is different from most saturated fats—it's made up of short- and medium-chain fatty acids, which your body can use very efficiently for energy. It doesn't contain any cholesterol, has a higher smoke point than vegetable oils (meaning it can tolerate higher heat before it begins to break down chemically and produce smoke), and won't go rancid like many other oils.

Higher-fat dairy. I used to buy all skim or low-fat dairy products, but now I buy the medium-fat or even full-fat products. I haven't gained any weight from it. I think consuming those fats helps your body regulate hormones better and also regulates your hunger levels. It also helps the body absorb the fat-soluble vitamins A and D, vitamins essential to the assimilation of protein. You may also find that eating 2 percent yogurt rather than fat-free, for instance, is more satisfying, so that you'll eat less and/or feel fuller longer.

> " Earlier this year, I was having a lot of gastrointestinal issues. Tracie Hittman Fountain suggested that I try going gluten-free for a couple of weeks. My doctor had tested me and said I was totally fine, but I tried giving it up for two weeks anyway. About three days in, I had so much energy I didn't know what to do with myself! By eight or nine days in, I was no longer suffering from any sort of gastrointestinal issues, so I stuck with it. I feel so much better now than I ever have in my life. I've never had energy like this."
>
> – Liz

Hydrolyzed gelatin. Gelatin is a very low-calorie source of protein you can mix into almost any liquid. Tracie recommends at least two tablespoons of hydrolyzed gelatin per day, not just for its protein content, but also because it can reduce inflammation and joint pain.

Olive oil. I like to use cold-pressed extra virgin olive oil, mainly for cold uses like salad dressings. With its lower smoke point, I really don't think it's great for cooking.

Go to Tracie's website, *itsyourplate.com*, to find more information about what to look for when buying gelatin and coconut oil, and links to purchase them online.

Meal Options

Breakfast (pick one)
Gluten-free
- 7 oz. Fagè Greek Yogurt with 1 T. honey or ½ c. fruit
- Smoothie: 1 c. organic milk (not skim), ¾ c. fruit, 2 T. hydrolyzed gelatin

Dairy-free
- Smoothie: ½ c. coconut milk, ½ c. water, ¾ c. fruit, 2 T. hydrolyzed gelatin
- Two hard-boiled eggs with a side of fruit
- ½ Ezekiel English muffin with egg cooked in coconut oil

Lunch (pick one)
Gluten-free
- Caprese salad*
- Amy's Cream of Tomato Soup with 1 T. gelatin added
- Greek salad (3 oz. pastured chicken, 1 oz. feta, tomato, cucumbers, and red onions with ½ T. olive oil)

Dairy-free
- Chicken salad* on cucumber and jicama slices
- Egg salad* on cucumber and tomato slices
- Tuna salad* with carrot sticks, cucumber, and tomato on one slice Ezekiel bread
- Amy's Lentil Soup with 1 T. gelatin added

Dinner (pick one)
Gluten-free
- Taco: 1 Food for Life sprouted corn tortilla, 3 oz. of taco meat, taco seasoning*, salsa, greens, and 1 oz. shredded cheese
- Crustless quiche*

Dairy-free
- Crock-Pot chicken*, with ½ sweet potato and ½ T. coconut oil
- Healthy stir-fry*
- 4 oz. grilled halibut, 1 c. zucchini cooked in ½ T. coconut oil

Desserts (for occasional treats)
Gluten-free
- 1 serving chocolate ricotta mousse*
- 1 serving fruit with yogurt sauce*
- 1 gluten-free coconut macaroon*

* See recipe.

Recipes

Crustless Veggie Quiche

6 servings, 250 calories each
C = 6g F = 19g P = 14g

Ingredients:
1 T. coconut oil
1 c. red peppers, chopped
1 c. zucchini, chopped
½ c. onion, chopped
6 oz. (1½ c.) rBGH-free cheese, shredded
6 farm-fresh eggs
½ tsp. sea salt
¼ tsp. black pepper
Ground nutmeg, to taste
⅛ tsp. garlic powder
1½ c. half-and-half
1 oz. (¼ c.) Parmesan cheese, grated

Instructions:
1. Preheat oven to 350°F.
2. Spread coconut oil in bottom of 9-inch baking dish.
3. Layer veggies and top with shredded cheese.
4. Beat eggs, half-and-half, salt, pepper, nutmeg, and garlic powder in medium bowl.
5. Pour over veggies and cheese.
6. Bake for 30 minutes; remove from oven and sprinkle with Parmesan cheese.
7. Return to oven and bake for 20 minutes longer, or until egg mix is set and top is slightly brown.
8. Remove from oven and let stand five minutes before serving.

Egg Salad

4 servings, 160 calories each
C = 2g F = 14g P = 10g

Ingredients:
6 large farm-fresh eggs
1-2 T. Wilderness Family mayonnaise or Greek yogurt
Salt and pepper
Tiny squeeze of lemon juice
2 stalks celery, chopped
½ bunch chives, chopped
Sea salt and pepper

Instructions:
1. Place the eggs in a pot and cover with cold water by a ½ -inch or so. Bring to a gentle boil.
2. Turn off the heat, cover, and let sit for seven to 12 minutes.
3. Have a big bowl of ice water ready, and when the eggs are done cooking, place them in it for about four minutes.
4. Crack and peel each egg. Place in a medium mixing bowl.
5. Add the mayonnaise and a couple generous pinches of salt and pepper. Now mash with a fork.
6. Don't overdo it. You want the egg mixture to have some texture.
7. Stir in the celery and chives. Taste and adjust the seasoning, adding more sea salt and pepper if needed.

Modified from:
101cookbooks.com/archives/001575.html

Tuna Salad

1 serving, 218 calories
C = 10g F = 6g P = 31g
Ingredients:
4 oz. tuna, canned in water
½ T. Wilderness Family mayonnaise or
Greek yogurt
6 grapes, sliced
½ medium carrot, shredded
Sea salt, to taste
Instructions:
Mix ingredients and enjoy.

Caprese Salad

6 servings, 252 calories each
C = 7g F = 17g P= 19g
Ingredients:
3 tomatoes, vine ripened, ¼-inch thick slices
1 lb. fresh rBGH-free mozzarella, ¼-inch slices
20 fresh basil leaves
2 T. olive oil, extra virgin for drizzling
1 T. balsamic vinegar
1 pinch sea salt and pepper
Instructions:
1. Layer alternating slices of tomatoes and
   mozzarella, adding a basil leaf between
   each, on a large, shallow platter.
2. Drizzle the salad with extra-virgin olive
   oil and vinegar, and season with salt and
   pepper to taste.

Crock-Pot Chicken with Herb Rub

Servings vary. 1 serving = 4 oz., 122 calories.
C = 0g F = 2g P = 26g
Ingredients:
One 3-4 lb. roasting chicken
Herb rub: Mix 1 tsp. each of the following
herbs: thyme, rosemary, oregano, seasoning
salt (MSG-free), and sea salt.
1 c. broth or stock
Instructions:
1. Rinse chicken under cold water.
   Remove any giblets and pat dry
   with paper towels.
2. In small bowl, combine herb rub
   ingredients.
3. Rub mixture on top and bottom of
   chicken.
4. Place in roaster or Crock-Pot with
   broth for three to four hours at
   225°F or on high.
5. Bones can be frozen to make bone
   broth at a later date.
*Recipe from Lynn Anderson of Anderson Farm,
Arkansaw, Wisconsin*

Chicken Salad

1 serving, 220 calories
C = 6g F = 13g P = 20g
Ingredients:
3 oz. pastured chicken, diced
1 T. Wilderness Family mayonnaise or
Greek yogurt
¼ c. celery, diced
Shredded carrots (optional)
Instructions:
Mix ingredients and enjoy.

Healthy Stir-Fry

4 servings, 340 calories each
C = 9g F = 17g P = 37g

Ingredients:

1 lb. grass-fed steak, sliced
¼ c. tamari (wheat-free soy sauce)
1-2 T. coconut oil
1 T. gelatin
1 c. beef broth
1 c. zucchini, sliced
½ c. bamboo shoots
1 c. peppers, chopped
1 c. carrots cut into matchsticks

Instructions:

1. Cut steak into strips and marinate in half the tamari sauce for 15 minutes.
2. Heat coconut oil in pan, then brown marinated steak.
3. While meat is browning, dissolve gelatin in beef broth by stirring gently.
4. Remove meat and add broth and gelatin to pan.
5. After broth is hot, add chopped veggies and sauté in broth mixture for five minutes.
6. Add beef and remaining tamari back to pan and stir until hot.
7. Serve in bowls and enjoy.

Taco Seasoning

Ingredients:

1 tsp. chili powder
1 tsp. paprika
⅛ - ¼ tsp. cayenne
¼ tsp. dried oregano
1 tsp. sea salt
½ tsp. ground cumin

Instructions:

1. Combine ingredients and mix until incorporated.
2. Add to 1 lb. of ground meat while cooking in a sauté pan. Taste when meat is fully cooked, and add more seasoning if desired.

Gluten-Free Coconut Macaroons

20 servings, 130 calories each
C = 10g F = 9g P = 1g

Ingredients:

6 egg whites
¼ tsp. sea salt
½ c. honey
1 T. vanilla extract
3 c. shredded coconut

Instructions:

1. In mixing bowl, whisk egg whites and salt until stiff.
2. Fold in honey, vanilla, and coconut.
3. Drop batter in rounded tablespoonfuls onto parchment-lined baking sheet.
4. Pinch each macaroon at top (like a Hershey's Kiss).
5. Bake at 350°F for 10-15 minutes, until lightly browned.

Chocolate Ricotta Mousse

8 servings, 160 calories each

C = 12g F = 10g P = 7g

Ingredients:

15 oz. container organic ricotta cheese (about 2 cups)

4 oz. semisweet chocolate, melted (such as Enjoy Life semisweet chocolate chips)

Fresh peppermint or spearmint for garnish (optional)

Instructions:

1. Bring ricotta to room temperature.
2. In a food processor, blend ricotta and melted chocolate until smooth.
3. The mousse can be refrigerated until ready to serve, up to two days.
4. Bring to room temperature before serving.
5. Garnish with a fresh mint leaf.

Fruit with Yogurt Sauce

6 servings, 150 calories each

C = 33g F = 2g P = 3g

Ingredients:

1 c. plain rBGH-free yogurt

2 T. honey

1½ tsp. grated lime rind

1 tsp. pure vanilla

3 c. pineapple, chopped

1 large peach, chopped

2 oranges, peeled and sectioned

2 kiwis, peeled and chopped

1 banana, sliced

Instructions:

1. Combine yogurt, honey, vanilla, and lime rind in a small bowl.
2. Combine the remaining fruit except the banana in a large bowl.
3. When ready to serve, add bananas to rest of the fruit and top with the yogurt sauce.

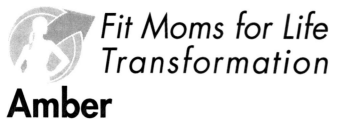

Fit Moms for Life Transformation

Amber

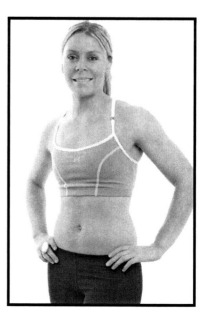

Amber started coming to my boot camps and took to heavy weight training right away. She got her body super-toned very quickly, fell in love with fitness, and is now one of my boot camp instructors.

When I first met her, I could tell there was a spark missing from her life, but she dove into boot camp headfirst and has made a 180-degree turnaround both internally and externally.

Amber's story: "My life is completely different from a year ago, when I was at my lowest. I was miserable with myself and my body, and it became a vicious cycle I could not get away from. All of my friendships were fading because I became reclusive and gave up on myself. But I knew that was not who I was. My life is much more rewarding and fun now with the confidence I've gained. I'm going forward with my dreams, and I've made great new friends through Dustin's program."

Amber's current goals: "I'm getting ready for a fitness modeling show and would like to do a triathlon at some point. Beyond fitness goals, I am working on a business plan for my own home decor and accessories store, which has been a dream of mine for a very long time!"

Amber's nutrition tips: "Get protein right away in the morning with breakfast, with a little bit of carbs and good fat. When I start my morning eating the right foods, I'm good to go the rest of the day."

Amber's exercise tips: "The thigh/butt area is definitely my work in progress. I've seen huge results with heavy lifting, sprint intervals, and jumping exercises."

Read more of Amber's story at *fitmomsforlife.com/amber.*

Amber, 30.
5'5", 125 pounds.
Amber went from a size 14 at her largest to a size 4, losing more than 25 pounds in just three months after she started coming to my boot camp

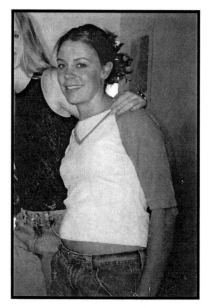

Fit Moms for Life Transformation

Jane

Jane has come a long way from the first day I met her, and literally looks like a different person now.

Jane's story: "I've never been super-fit, but never very overweight. I always liked being active, but never found a way to incorporate exercise into my life in a really reliable way, especially as life got busier and busier. The realization that my 50th birthday was coming up was my motivation to really focus and get in shape. I started doing Dustin's boot camp. At first I didn't take it that seriously, but as my birthday got closer, I started to put in a lot more effort and addressed my eating. I didn't want to do something temporary, but wanted to figure out how to live in a healthier way. I already had a lot of good habits, so I just had to figure out how to cement those and minimize the bad stuff.

"I recently achieved my goal of doing 50 push-ups—and I think I could probably do more if I really pushed myself. I also dropped a minute and a half off the time it takes me to sprint up the hill we run at boot camp. It took me six minutes the first time I ever did it, and I got below four and a half last summer.

"I think my kids are really proud of me, which is nice. My daughter said to me the other day, 'Your arms look like Michelle Obama's, but better.' They've always been proud of me for other things, but they're really conscious of how I have worked toward something and made it fit into our lives without making it rule our lives."

Jane's nutrition tips: "Go to farmer's markets. Everything looks so good at a farmer's market; it's really appealing. And you feel a connection and an enthusiasm about it, and I think that makes you more inclined to eat those healthy foods. Buying the same thing at the grocery store, even if it's organic or locally grown, just doesn't have the same feel."

Read more of Jane's story at *fitmomsforlife.com/jane.*

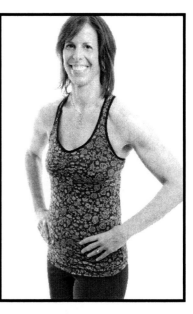

Jane, 50, mother of three. 5'10", 144 pounds. Jane went from a size 10 to a size 6 through intense workouts and eating well.

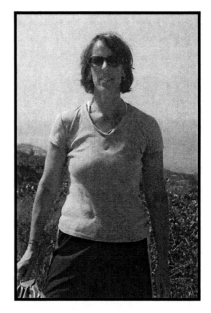

Making It Work

I hope that the rules I described in the last chapter made sense to you, and the meal ideas and recipes gave you a sense of how to put the rules into practice. In this chapter, I want to share tips and ideas that have worked for me and for my clients to make this way of eating into a sustainable lifestyle.

It's really about being a knowledgeable consumer and eater, and being accountable for what goes into your mouth. Once you focus on it for a long enough time, you'll undo some of your bad habits and create new, healthy ones, and it will become second nature. Until that happens, for those first few weeks or months—or even up to a year for some people—you've really got to be diligent. You don't want to slip into your old patterns, and you want to catch yourself and get back on track quickly if that does happen. All your hard work is definitely going to pay off. You're going to feel better. You're going to lose weight, if that's your goal. You'll have a tighter, fitter body. The long-term bonus is that eating healthy and being fit significantly decreases your odds of developing many serious diseases.

Besides the meal plans and tips I share in this book, I also recommend checking out my friend Isabel De Los Rios' website, *thedietsolutionprogram.com*. Her online diet book has helped hundreds of thousands of people from nearly every country in the world.

Tips for Putting It Into Practice
Plan ahead. I think the biggest difference between eating the way I recommend and eating the way most people eat is active planning and preparation. You've already read a little bit about this in Chapter 5 (Rule 14: "Be prepared"), but I can't stress it enough. You might feel overwhelmed thinking that it's going to take you a lot of extra time, but if you do this carefully, you will probably spend the same amount of time you're spending on food preparation now, maybe even less. I'm

talking about 10 or 15 minutes in the evening to prep some things for the next day, and/or maybe three hours on a Sunday to make things you'll use in your meals for the rest of the week. You'll be so much more efficient putting meals together when you've done that preparation. Even more important, you won't be caught in situations where you're tempted to make unhealthy choices.

Cook in large quantities. Cooking things in larger quantities is one of your biggest time-savers and a great way to be prepared. In addition to saving you energy, it will also save you money on groceries (because you can buy things on sale or in bulk). So, cook twice as much (or three times as much, or more) as you need for one meal, and put enough for another meal in a reusable container or a freezer bag in the refrigerator or freezer. When it's time to use it, you can warm it up, and you'll have a fresh, healthy meal without all the preservatives you'd get in a frozen meal from the store. Even if you're not freezing whole meals, you can cook something like brown rice in huge quantities, and freeze individual portion sizes or the amount your family uses for dinner, so you can grab that when you're short on time.

> *Before I leave the house in the morning I make my kids' lunches, and then I also make my lunch and snacks. I bring an apple and a piece of string cheese to work, and sometimes a protein shake. And then maybe a salad or a healthy sandwich for lunch. That keeps me out of the office kitchen, which can be a dangerous place! It also keeps me out of restaurants where I might make unhealthy choices."*
>
> – Kelly

Time your nutrition around exercise. There's been a lot of research in the last 10 years about nutrient timing with exercise. I'll just summarize it here. (If you're interested in this subject at a deeper level, I recommend the book *Nutrient Timing* by John Ivy and Robert Portman.) Basically, your body responds differently to certain nutrients during and after your workout than at other times throughout the day.

One of the big questions is whether you should work out on an empty stomach. There are conflicting beliefs out there, and research to support both approaches. Some people say that doing cardio and/or lifting weights on an empty stomach will burn more fat. Other people say you shouldn't do that. They argue that you should consume at least a small amount of food, because if you don't have sugar in your body to fuel the workout, your body will break down muscle to get the fuel it needs. My belief is that you should have at least a little bit of food before exercising. You're going to be able to work out harder and more intensely if you have a little boost of energy in your body, even if it is only 100 calories. So that's what I do, but I suggest you try both ways and see what works best for you.

I generally tell people to eat 10 to 20 grams of protein and 15 to 20 grams of carbs within the 30 minutes before they work out. Those carbs should be simple sugars, like you find in fruit. I don't recommend simple sugars much throughout the rest of the day, but before and after working out are the two times I do. You should have simple sugars and protein, which will give your body energy and nutrients right before you exercise, whether you're doing cardio or strength training.

I'm not a big fan of juice, but if you're going to drink it, before a workout would be the time to do it, along with some protein. Personally, I prefer to use protein drinks before I work out. I think it's the easiest thing to do. For instance, I usually have a little bit of milk (which also provides carbs) with a whey protein powder. (See page 87 for information about which supplements I use and why.) Whey protein breaks down very fast in your body, so it's a great way to get protein circulating through the bloodstream and into your muscles while you're working out. Greek yogurt is another good option—it has some whey protein in it. Throw in some berries or a piece of fruit, which are great sources of simple sugars.

What's even more important is what you eat after your workout. You have about a 45-minute window when your muscles are up to 400 percent more receptive than usual for sugar and especially protein.[1] You want to get protein into the muscles as quickly as possible to start the rebuilding and repairing process after you've worked out. Researchers have found that the most efficient way to do that is by having the protein carried into the bloodstream by sugar. The ratio that they've found to be most effective at this point is about a 2:1 or 3:1 ratio of sugar to protein. For a woman, a good guideline is to get about 15 grams of protein and about 30 grams of carbs. If you're significantly overweight, you might want to cut the carbs back a little bit. Otherwise, you could go up to as much as 45 grams of carbs with 15 grams of protein.

We're looking for simple sugars, just as we did before the workout. If you eat a complex carb like brown rice or whole wheat, that takes awhile to break down in your stomach, and that's time wasted as far as the muscle recovery process is concerned. This is another great time to incorporate fruit into your diet. Post-workout is also another good time for a protein drink, because you're going to get good protein and sugars.

Of course, you'll find formulated pre-workout and post-workout drinks, which can work too. I have links to some good ones on my website. Just remember, there's nothing magical about a powder like that. It just already has the right amount of nutrients in it, so it saves you some of the thinking and preparation time.

Be smart about eating out. People always have a lot of questions about how they can continue to eat meals out when they're following my program. The simple answer is to eat out as little as possible. Most restaurant food is not good for you, unfortunately. But you can go into a restaurant with some great strategies to keep your meal as healthy as possible.

The most important thing to do is to educate yourself about what's available wherever you will be eating. The restaurant edition of *Eat This, Not That*, by David Zinczenko and Matt Goulding, is a

---

1 Rasmussen, et al. "An Oral Essential Amino Acid-Carbohydrate Supplement Enhances Muscle Protein Anabolism after Resistance Exercise." Journal of Applied Physiology 88 (2000): 386-92.

great place to start. Sometimes you don't have a choice about where you go, but if you know where you're going in advance, you can usually look it up in a book like that, or go to the restaurant's website and find at least the calories in each menu item. Even with all the time I've spent learning about nutrition, I've been surprised to discover that a dish I thought was pretty healthy or low-calorie was actually less healthy than something I thought was really bad for me. Take a look at whatever nutritional information you can find.

There are a few practical things you can do while you're at a restaurant, too.

Skip the bread or chips. Many restaurants serve bread or chips before the meal. I love that stuff and, of course, it's tempting to eat the whole basket—especially because it's free, right? But ask your server not to bring it out at all. You won't even miss it, and it's a lot easier than letting it sit there calling your name from the corner of the table. Just say no from the start.

Stick to the main course. Don't eat appetizers. The meal itself will be big enough. It will provide enough calories and enough energy. Don't drink soda. Just drink water. If you're going to have a glass of wine, get it with your meal. But for the most part, just drink water. This is also a big money-saver if you make it into a habit for your whole family, because restaurant soda is so expensive. Don't get dessert, because the entrée is providing all the energy you need.

Keep your portions under control. If you're with your husband, significant other, or a friend, I suggest splitting an entrée. Amazingly, restaurant portion sizes are sometimes four to five times larger than what would be considered a healthy portion. So you can get a big meal and split it in half, and that should be about the right calorie range for the meal. Another option is to get the full meal, but ask for a take-home container right away, and put half of it away to take home for lunch the next day. You can also check the appetizer menu for any healthy options, which will come in a more realistic portion size. Just ask for it to be brought out at the same time as everyone else's dinner.

Don't be shy about being very particular when you order. You're paying the restaurant to make the food the way you want it. The nicer the restaurant, the more successful your requests for changes or substitutions may be. You can ask for steamed vegetables on the side instead of something deep-fried. You can ask them to steam your fish or ask them to cook your meat without fat or oil, or without additional salt.

This may be different from what you are familiar with when you eat out, but by becoming aware, skipping the extras, and making some substitutions, you can save yourself thousands of calories when dining in a restaurant. You won't be changing the experience of the meal or your night out, but you can keep it from setting you back a week in your weight loss! Of course, if it's your anniversary or your birthday, you might choose to go all out and order whatever you want. Just don't make that a regular thing. The more frequently you eat out, the more important these strategies will be to stay on track.

If you have friends in your area who are also trying to eat better, share tips about restaurants that have healthy options and those that don't. Ask around, and share what you learn!

Don't clean your kids' plates. I know this is a big one for a lot of moms. They eat their healthy meal in the right portion sizes, and then they clean their kids' plates at the end of the meal. Sound familiar? If you have two kids and you do that at several meals a day, you might add 300 to 500 calories to your day! I think many moms believe that they shouldn't waste any food, so they can't bring themselves to throw away what the kids didn't eat. My recommendation is to either start giving your kids smaller portion sizes—they can always take seconds if they eat what you give them—or plan on their leftovers being part of your meal, so that you don't end up overeating. Other options would be to throw away their uneaten food or save it for later.

> *One of the biggest changes I've made is to realize that my daughter's food is her food. At restaurants, I was ordering her french fries and eating half of them."*
> – Aimee

Healthy Snack Ideas

When you're eating four to six times a day, you need some flexibility and variety to put together good meals and snacks. (Some people like to eat roughly the same amount each time they eat, but having some larger meals with smaller snacks in between is fine, too.) I'll throw out a few ideas here, and then you'll see a list of snacks that I recommend on page 86. Most of these snacks are in the 50- to 200-calorie range. None of them have carbs by themselves, most of them are easy to transport, and many are a hit with kids.

A great approach is to combine a carb with a protein. One of the easiest ways to do this is to combine fruit with cheese. Cheese has some protein in it and some fat. As long as you watch your portion size, it'll be a healthy amount of fat. I like to use string cheese because it's already portioned for you and it's very easy to carry. An apple and a string cheese make a terrific snack. A banana and cheese work too, but bananas are a bit higher in sugar, so I save those for right before or after a workout. You can always go with a lean meat for your protein. Try a couple of slices of deli meat combined with a piece of fruit or a slice of whole-grain bread.

> *It's easier than you think it is. Yes, it is easy to grab a bag of Doritos and open them up and serve them as a snack. But it is also easy to grab a bag of pretzels and hummus to dip them in."*
> – Jody

Another healthy option for a small snack is nuts. Best choices would be almonds, walnuts, sunflower seeds, or pistachios. They give you fat and protein together. You want to get raw, unsalted nuts (roasting breaks down the quality of the fat). Watch your portion size to be sure you aren't overdoing the fat or the calories! Try weighing an ounce of nuts to get a sense of portion size. Plain regular or

Greek yogurt is a perfect snack on its own or with some fruit—it provides a nice level of fat, protein, and a bit of natural carbs.

I like to use protein drinks for my snacks. There are several ways to make protein drinks, and I'll share my favorite with you. I use 100 percent whey protein powder and combine it with frozen berries and either water or milk. I like to make two servings in the morning and have one at midmorning and one in the afternoon. It helps fill me up and keeps me going until my next bigger meal.

Healthy Snack Ideas

Nuts or seeds and fruit (gluten- and dairy-free). For example:
- 2 T. raw pecans + ½ c. unsweetened applesauce.
- 2 T. raw cashews + ½ c. grapes.
- 12 raw almonds + 1 c. sliced mango or an apple.
- 2 T. pumpkin (pepitas) or sunflower seeds + 2 c. melon.

Plain yogurt with additions (gluten-free). For example:
- ½ c. plain yogurt + 1 c. berries + 1 T. non-sugar jam.
- ½ c. plain yogurt + 1 T. natural peanut butter + ¼ sliced banana.

Cheese and fruit/vegetables (gluten-free). For example:
- 1-1.5 oz. white cheese + 1 medium pear.
- 1 string cheese + 1 kiwi.
- 1 oz. feta cheese + ½ c. unsweetened applesauce or sliced peaches.
- String cheese + 1 c. sliced cucumber.

Vegetables and hummus (gluten- and dairy-free). For example:
- 1 c. sliced red or green peppers + ¼ c. hummus (made with olive oil).
- 1 c. mixed jicama sticks and carrot sticks + ¼ c. hummus (made with olive oil).

Bread with protein/fat (can be dairy-free). For example:
- 1 slice whole-grain or sprouted grain bread + string cheese.
- 1 slice whole-grain or sprouted grain toast + 1 hardboiled egg + 1 tsp. non-sugar jam.
- 1 slice whole-grain or sprouted grain bread + can of tuna.

Cottage cheese with fruit (gluten-free). For example:
- ½ c. cottage cheese + ½ c. unsweetened applesauce.
- ½ c. cottage cheese + ½ c. unsweetened pineapple.
- ½ c. cottage cheese + 1 medium orange.

Other
- 10 oz. glass of grass-fed or organic milk (gluten-free).
- ½ c. unsweetened applesauce + 2 T. gelatin (mixed in) (gluten- and dairy-free).
- Hot herbal or green tea + 1 T. gelatin + ½ T. coconut oil + ½ T. honey (gluten- and dairy-free).

Protein Drinks and Other Supplements

I'm not an expert in supplements, but I get a lot of questions about them, so I want to say a little bit about it here. First of all, most people who ask about supplements are looking for the magic pill that's going to help them lose massive amounts of weight. Most of those "increase your metabolism" pills and "fat burner" supplements seem to get pulled off the market at some point, either because they aren't effective or because they're unsafe. I don't use "magic pill" supplements, and I don't recommend them. The bottom line is that you have to eat well and focus on real food. If you're eating the right foods and you can afford to try supplements with some of your income, that's fine. But I wouldn't want to see you spending money that you could be spending on higher-quality food for yourself and your family on supplements.

That's not to say that I don't think supplementation can be beneficial. In some situations, it is very beneficial. So I'll run through the ones I've found that research shows to be effective, and the ones that I use myself. You can see more about all of these at *fitmomsforlife.com/supplements*.

First of all, the protein drinks I have most every day can be considered supplemental, and I recommend them—not because protein drinks are some magical formula, but because it's an easy, convenient way to increase your protein intake. Many people have difficulty getting in enough protein throughout the day, and protein drinks can be a big help. When you're looking for protein powder, I recommend going for a 100 percent whey protein. Since there are some big questions about how healthy processed soy is for our bodies, you definitely don't want a soy-based protein powder. If you are lactose-intolerant, rice protein would be the next best substitute. The other important thing is to get one that doesn't have fake sugars in it. It will probably be sweetened with something like stevia, which is natural. (Steer clear of the ones with high levels of sugar, which are often labeled "weight gainer.") What I look for is 15 to 20 grams of protein per serving, and maybe 1 to 4 grams of fat. That makes for about 120 calories per serving, plus whatever you add to it, which will fill you up and give you the right nutrients between meals.

I also use an omega-3 fish oil and krill oil supplement. The research out there about how beneficial and important omega-3s and omega-6s are is staggering. I also take a multivitamin every day. I guess I do that more out of faith that it's working than because I can feel the results. The way soil conditions are these days, even when we do our best to eat as much whole food and as naturally as we can, there are likely going to be some deficiencies in our diet. I use the multivitamin to make up for those deficiencies.

Grocery Shopping Strategies

I occasionally offer grocery store tours for my clients in Madison, Wisconsin, where I live. I love to do them because it really opens people's eyes about what is in the foods they're eating, and what food producers and stores are doing to try to steer our decisions in some pretty unhealthy directions. (By the way, a great resource for more information like this is *Food, Inc.* It's a brilliant documentary about where your food comes from and some of the politics behind food policy in America today. It is a powerful movie that will definitely make you want to change some of your eating decisions.) So here are some tips for becoming an educated consumer and a good shopper for healthy food.

Read labels. Give yourself the time to look closely at ingredient labels on your next trip to buy groceries. (If you can, leave the kids at home so you can concentrate!) On my grocery store tours, moms in particular get upset when they see what's actually in some of the foods they buy for their kids. Whatever it says on the front of the package to make the food sound healthy is often a lie. The first thing I look at is the length of the ingredient list and the number of ingredients. Let's say you're comparing five or six boxes of breakfast cereal. Without

> " I've learned so much about being careful of exactly what is in food. So now I'm really thorough on reading labels. It's amazing to me how many ingredients there can be in cottage cheese, and how many different versions of cottage cheese are in the store."
> – Tina

even reading the ingredients themselves, I can tell you that the one with the shortest ingredient list is probably the best one for you. The shorter list means it has a smaller number of ingredients and fewer of those chemical additives with the really long, unpronounceable names. The number of ingredients tells you a lot about how processed something is. In breads, for example, the difference is amazing between something like Ezekiel bread (a sprouted grain bread you can find in the frozen section), with five to eight ingredients, and a more conventional bread, which probably has 30 or 40, a lot of them chemicals. Think about how many ingredients you would need to make bread at home—not many. So why do they need so many ingredients to make the bread for sale at the store?

As far as actually reading an ingredient list goes, you need to know that ingredients are listed in order of amount, measured by weight. So the first ingredient on the list is the most prevalent, and the first five or six usually make up the bulk of the product. If you're looking for something with whole grains, you want the whole grain to be the first ingredient, not number 17, after all kinds of more processed ingredients. Then you want to look for ingredients that you can pronounce and that you can recognize as food. Is this product made from whole foods and components of whole foods, or are they adding a lot of different food colorings or preservatives? Are there partially hydrogenated oils and other things that contain trans fats?

Shop the perimeter. One of the best strategies to get healthy foods at a grocery store is to stick to the edges of the store and steer clear of the aisles in the middle. All your fresh produce and natural foods are around the edges. Most stores start with the fruits and vegetables, which you want to get a lot of. As you walk around, you'll get to the dairy section, where you want to get milk, cheese, cottage cheese, and yogurt (I like plain Greek yogurt with its higher protein content and no added sweeteners). Then you get to the meat section, where I recommend you buy lean products like chicken and turkey. Sticking to the perimeter, you'll eventually arrive at the freezer section. Frozen vegetables and fruits are great, especially for things that aren't in season or aren't grown in your region. Those fruits and vegetables are actually frozen at the peak of freshness, so they can be better for you than the "fresh" stuff that's been shipped from halfway around the world, which was possibly packed when it was still unripe and ripened with chemicals along the way. Once you've covered all of that, there aren't many aisles you actually need to go down.

> " *Read the labels when you go to the store. I don't think people realize how much bad stuff is put in packaged and processed foods. The label might say 'low fat,' for example, but if you really look at the ingredients, you'll see it's not good for you."*
>
> – Patrice

Make a list and stick to it. Have a list with you, so that you aren't tempted to impulse-buy junk food just because it looks or sounds good. If you've already planned your meals for the week, you should know what you need. Even if you haven't planned all your meals, make a list of the healthy ingredients you want to have on hand for the week.

Don't shop hungry. I've noticed that I'm much more likely to buy something unhealthy if I'm really hungry when I go shopping. Go right after you've eaten a good meal and you'll be less tempted by everything you see.

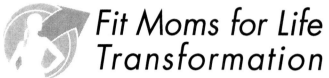

Fit Moms for Life Transformation

Crystal

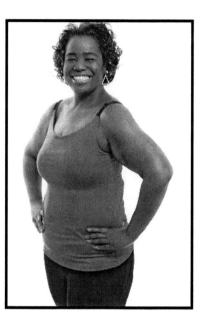

When I met Crystal, I was immediately struck by her contagious laugh and great personality. But she was carrying so much weight that it was going to cause serious health problems down the road. She is in the process of making an amazing transformation through my program.

Crystal's story: "When I started Fit Fun Boot Camps, I weighed 279 pounds. I had tried different fitness and nutritional approaches before, but none really stuck. I tried a three-week trial of boot camp. My weight didn't budge a lot in those first three weeks, but I noticed some internal changes regarding energy, my outlook on life, and a reduction in stress level. So I decided to keep doing it, and it changed my life.

"I've always been confident in who I am. Even when I was heavier, I tried to put my best foot forward. But I think by losing the weight, I'm even more confident in who I am internally. I'm okay with who I am and with putting myself out there.

"When I began my weight-loss journey, I never really considered that I might inspire other people to improve their health and their lives. But a lot of my friends and family look at me and say, 'I want to do it, too!' So that is inspiring me to help others."

Crystal's current goals: "My goal size is probably about a size 8 or so. But it is difficult to say, because for me it is not so much the dress size, as it's what my body can do."

Crystal's exercise tips: "Your body can do so much more than you give it credit for. Every time you say, 'I'm tired,' if you push yourself one more step or take one more breath or do one more rep—you can do it. And in the end you push yourself further than you thought you could go."

Crystal's advice to you: "You might be unhappy about where you are, but don't let that define who you are. Think about where you want to be. Think about the goals you need to make to get there, and develop a support system to help you. Think about the lifestyle you want to have, and let that be your motivation."

Read more of Crystal's story at *fitmomsforlife.com/crystal.*

Crystal, 28.
5'3", 189 pounds.
Crystal lost 90 pounds, went from a size 22 to a size 12, took 14 inches off her waist in 13 months, and is still going strong.

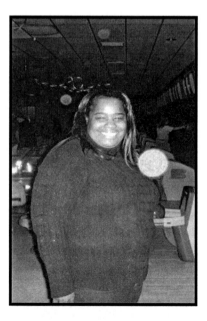

Fit Moms for Life Transformation

Katy

Katy started coming to MamaTone when her youngest was just six weeks old, and she has refused to let any excuses get in her way. She's made an amazing physical transformation and gained confidence in herself.

Katy's story: "I ran cross-country in high school and stayed fit that way. But when I went to college, got married, and had kids, I kind of gave up on fitness. After each kid, I tried to work out. But I kept saying to myself, "I'm going to have another one. What difference does it make if I get back in shape?" After the third one, I knew I was done having kids, so I had to finally do something. That's when I found Dustin and started going to MamaTone.

"Along with the physical changes, I'd definitely say I'm more self-confident now. I used to kind of hide in the crowd. I'm much more confident now about going places and meeting new people, and I am definitely more outgoing. Also, I'm a stay-at-home mom, and it's much easier to keep up with my kids now. I actually play with them a lot more. Last summer we went outside more than normal and played in the park, and I run around with them a lot more. They've noticed, too."

Katy's nutrition tips: "One: Read the labels. I had never read a label before. I always shopped by what was the cheapest. Now I read all the ingredients, and if I don't understand what's in it, I don't buy it, because it can't be good. Two: The protein-carb combo is great, especially for snacks. If you grab a protein and a carb, it definitely holds you over better than one or the other. And you're not hungry all the time, which is the downfall of any diet. Three: I have a major sweet tooth, so a little piece of dark chocolate or some other little sweet after dinner makes me feel like I'm not completely missing out on enjoying food."

Katy's advice to you: "You can get back in shape. This isn't the way it has to be forever. Sometimes it seems impossible, but it's not. You just need to find the right tools and what works for you."

Read more of Katy's story at *fitmomsforlife.com/katy.*

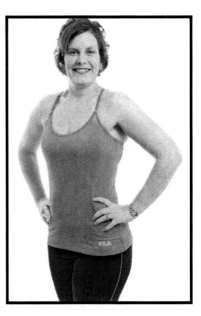

Katy, 33, mother of three.
5'7", 136 pounds.
Katy lost 48 pounds and
nine inches from her waist,
and went from 41 percent
body fat to 24 percent.

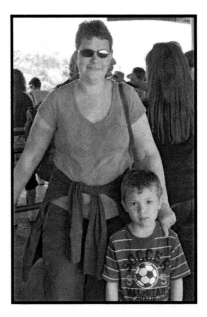

STRENGTH AND BURST TRAINING: MOVING TO BE FIT FOR LIFE

"Dustin's program takes the guesswork out of exercising. It takes the pressure off of you because you have somebody who's an expert telling you what you need to do to get results—and it works." – Tiffany

"It's very heartening when you start to see muscles, like all of a sudden. It's like you're passing the mirror and you go, 'Oh my God. Really? Is that my shoulder? Are you serious?' And then you ask strangers to feel how hard your shoulder is." – Aimee

One of my taglines is "Keep Moving," because I think exercise is one of the most important contributors to health, fitness, and general well-being. If you have a body that can move, I think you should get off your butt and use it so that it will continue to serve you well.

A hundred years ago, no one was recommending strength training or any sort of exercise for the sake of staying healthy, because people were very active and most were fit. A lot of people lived on farms, where they did a lot of carrying and pushing and basically moved all day long. Many women carried heavy buckets and did laundry by hand. There was a lot of manual labor in most people's lives. Today, most Americans live more sedentary lives. You might spend a lot of time chasing your kids around and picking them up, but that isn't much work in a physical sense. Most of us are not really working all of our body parts, which is why we need to seek out ways to challenge our bodies, burn calories, and build our muscles.

In this section, I'm going to introduce you to my exercise program. My program focuses on efficiency and effectiveness, so that you can challenge your body and achieve your goals without spending hours a day working out. First, I'll explain the benefits of strength training and describe what kind of exercises you should be doing. Then, I'll describe burst training—you'll be shocked at how little time you can spend on cardio if you do it intensely enough. Finally, I'll help you establish your own exercise routine and share a sample workout from one of my *Fit Moms for Life* DVDs.

7

Lifting in Order to Tone

In the 1980s and 1990s, skinny was in. That emaciated "skin and bones" look was never healthy, but it was definitely trendy. Now I think a fit, healthy, toned-looking body is starting to be the "in" thing. That's fantastic, because it's actually healthy—and it's very empowering for women. I hear from so many moms who are doing my programs, saying they just feel good. They feel strong and powerful with the extra strength they've gained through strength training. They feel ready to take on other challenges in their lives because they've discovered a strength they didn't know they had. Strength training is the first step in that journey, and I'm going to teach you how to build your strength using challenging weights.

> " I feel sexier. I feel more confident. I am proud to show my shoulders and my arms. I have the right to bare arms! There is almost like a sisterhood with the women who lift weights."
>
> – Karen B.

My friend Alwyn Cosgrove is a co-author of a great book titled *The New Rules of Lifting for Women: Lift Like a Man, Look Like a Goddess*. I highly recommend this book for even more in-depth reading on lifting weights. Alwyn's wife Rachel also has an awesome book called *The Female Body Breakthrough* which talks significantly about how and why resistance training is essential for women.

Why Strength Training Is Important for Women

Toning. The biggest reason I recommend strength training is because of its toning effect. A lot of women think they're going to get big and bulky by lifting weights, but that's just not the case. Women have between 15 to 30 times less testosterone than men, which really limits their ability to gain muscle. So unless a woman is shooting up with steroids, she's not going to get bulky. Even if she were within the very small percentage of the population who have an athletic build and are genetically more inclined to put on muscle, a woman would have to work extremely hard at lifting and have a higher-calorie diet to gain a serious amount of muscle. As you flip through this book and look at the success stories, you won't see a woman with "bulky" muscles—and all of these women do significant strength training. When women lift weights, their muscles actually become more defined and toned, without getting bigger. They get sleek and strong arms, like Michelle Obama's or Kelly Ripa's. Everyone wants that strong, lean, muscular look. You can only get that look with strength training.

> " The thing with the weight training that I love is I actually have muscle tone, which I have never had before in my 37 years. It's nice when I look at my arms and they are hard. They are nice, hard, solid muscular arms."
> – Jody

After-burn. Another big benefit of strength training is the after-burn effect of the workouts. We all like to see that "calories burned" number going higher and higher on the treadmill. In fact, you burn about the same number of calories in a session of treadmill running as you do in a session of circuit strength training, but when we look at what happens after the workout, strength training takes the lead. "Excess post-exercise oxygen consumption"—or after-burn, as most people call it—is the boost in calories burned following an intense workout. Studies in the 1980s and 1990s convinced everyone that cardio was the best way to burn fat, but they didn't take after-burn into account. More recent studies have looked at how your metabolism changes over the 48 hours from when you start exercising. They found that you burn a significant number of additional calories in the 48 hours after a strength training session. The after-burn is much lower for cardio. Let's say you do a strength training routine that burns 250 calories in 30 minutes. Another time, you run for 30 minutes and burn 300 calories. At first glance, it looks like the strength training burned fewer calories. But look at the after-burn. In the 48 hours after running, you're going to burn an extra 50 to 100 calories beyond what you normally would. However, after the strength training session, you'll burn an extra 200 to 400 calories in the next 48 hours. You're burning 350 to 400 total calories with the run, and 450 to 650 total calories with the strength training.

> " Strength training is the best thing you can do for your body. I have really noticed, especially as I get older and it was starting to slow down, that my metabolism picked up again when I started strength training. There have been times I can hardly eat enough to keep up, which is something I never thought I would say. I would never, ever go without strength training again."
> – Karen E.

Fat-burning state. There is also some interesting research about the type of fuel your body uses when you do different types of exercise. At this point we don't really know why this happens, but the body seems to go into a fat-burning state during and after strength training. Conversely, it is more likely to be in a sugar-burning or carb-burning state with cardio.

Bone density. Strength training is the best way to increase bone density from an exercise standpoint. It's pretty amazing what it's able to do. I have studied osteopenia (low bone mineral density) and osteoporosis (very low bone mineral density) extensively. Just to give you a quick overview, women have until about the age of 25 or 30 to maximize their bone density. That's why

> *You can always get there, but it's a lot easier to start now and to have the strong muscles and bones that will help in your older years."*
>
> – Donna

it's really important that adolescent girls and young women start to strength train, because that's when you're going to build your bone density up as much as you can. After the age of 30, your goal is not to lose bone density. Most women don't see too much of a decline in their thirties and forties, but once they hit menopause and don't have estrogen helping keep their bones strong, they see a big decline in bone density. The majority of women who live past 50 will have osteoporosis or osteopenia, with about 40 percent suffering an osteoporotic fracture in their lifetimes.[1] It's a huge problem, with serious consequences for your quality of life as you get older. So what can be done? Research has shown that women who have lost a lot of bone density or even just started the decline after menopause were able to increase their bone density by 1 or 2 percent through strength training. Now, that's not a big jump, but since you'd otherwise see big declines, being able to stabilize bone density and even increase it somewhat is vital.

Strength training is very good for bone density because it loads the bones and muscles with weight. And in a good strength training program where you're working all the parts of your body, you'll improve bone strength throughout your body. Other types of exercise just don't get that effect. For example, running is very joint-specific. It will put a load on the hip area, but it won't benefit the bones in the rest of your body. Things like walking, biking, or swimming that are lower-impact do very little for your bone density.

Cardiovascular benefits. Strength training can also have cardiovascular benefits if you follow my program and train the way I'm going to teach you. My program gets your heart rate very high, similar to cardio, and of course that brings the benefits of cardiovascular health and a stronger heart. The heart has to pump the blood a lot harder during strength training. The walls of the heart actually increase in size over time, which positively affects the transportation of oxygen, nutrients, and minerals through the body. My client Becky, who is unable to use her legs for any traditional cardiovascular exercise, has

> *I hadn't run a mile since I was in high school, but I decided to see what would happen if I tried to run on the treadmill. I ran a mile, and I was barely out of breath! We never run a mile in boot camp, but you're just strengthening your heart and the rest of your body, and that carries over into so many other things."*
>
> – Tina

1 Looker, A.C., et al. "Prevalence of Low Femoral Bone Density in Older U.S. Adults from NHANES III." Journal of Bone and Mineral Research 12.11 (1997): 1761-68.

improved her overall fitness through strength training alone. She doesn't take any breaks between strength training exercises, so she keeps her heart rate high throughout her workout, and that has been enough to improve her cardiovascular endurance.

Myths about Strength Training

"Strength training will make me bulk up." I've explained why this is not true. The pictures of my clients in this book, who all do strength training on a regular basis, show that strength training does not mean "bulking up." Abby can bench press 130 pounds and squat 300—and she is not remotely bulky, as you can see on page 31.

"Steady-state cardio is the best way to burn fat." I believe that steady-state cardio actually makes people fat, and I will explain why in the next chapter. Strength training burns more calories than cardio, puts your body in fat-burning mode, and helps raise your metabolism. It is a much better way to burn fat than endless cardio.

"Strength training is dangerous." Any time you move your body, there's a risk that you could get hurt. If you do any kind of exercise for long enough, you will probably experience some sort of injury. But I would argue that if you're sedentary and not doing any exercise, you're more likely to hurt yourself doing something like vacuuming, coughing, or picking up your child—and you're more likely to face serious health problems in the long term that limit your mobility or your ability to use your body at all. Personally, I'd rather face the occasional minor injury. And I don't believe strength training is any riskier than other forms of exercise. You have to use weights you can control and do your lifting with good form. (You can ask a trainer or a friend to assess your form. If you're working out alone to a DVD, pause it to watch the form very closely, and look in a mirror to see if you're getting it right.) Please don't use the fear of injury as an excuse not to start a program that could change your life.

Sustained weight loss. My program is designed to help you lose weight and keep it off—and strength training is critical for that to happen. You've probably seen people lose weight by eating a very calorie-restricted diet and running or doing a lot of cardio. Maybe you've even done it yourself. It can be effective in the short term because if you're not eating very many calories and you're exercising, you're going to lose body fat. But unfortunately, without enough calories, your body is tapping into muscles to get the sugar it needs to do the exercise. As you lose muscle,

> Once I started to lose a couple of pounds each week, it was like, 'OK, now I can do this.' At the beginning, when you don't lose anything, it's hard."
> – Katy

your basal metabolic rate drops—remember, muscle is very metabolically active and burns a lot of calories. To keep losing weight or even maintain your weight at that point, you have to eat fewer and fewer calories or exercise more and more. It's a nasty cycle. It's the reason so many people gain weight back on other programs, when they get sick of not eating enough or they can't increase their exercise anymore. What I see with my clients is consistent weight loss that can be maintained because they are building muscle and raising their metabolism over time through strength training. At the same time, they're eating fewer calories than they used to, but not depriving themselves. The weight loss might be a little slower at first, but it sticks better.

Structuring Your Workout

The most important things you want to do with strength training are work your entire body and build muscle (which will help you raise your metabolism, burn more calories, and raise your heart rate while you're lifting). That means you want to work the largest muscles the most, because that will stimulate the greatest number of muscle fibers. I see a lot of women who just focus on smaller muscle groups, like the biceps, because that's where they want to see the muscle definition. But without the larger muscles helping to burn more calories, you aren't going to lose the fat that's obscuring the biceps and get all the other benefits of strength training. The best advice I can give you is to work your larger muscle groups the most.

> " A lot of people are like, 'Oh, you're going to get a bad knee or get a bad this or a bad that by doing these types of physical workouts.' But I think you get those bad knees when you don't do the workouts."
>
> – Trish

In your lower body, that means working the muscles in your upper legs and butt. Always incorporate some sort of squat; some sort of lunge; some sort of step-up; some sort of dead lift; and a hip-raise motion to work the hamstrings and glutes. The sample workout in Chapter 9 includes examples of these types of exercises. You can throw in some calf raises once in a while, but that's a smaller muscle group, so I wouldn't focus on those too much.

In the upper body, you need to focus on your back and shoulders as the largest muscle groups. That means you want to include some sort of pushing exercise like a push-up or a bench press; some sort of overhead pressing exercise; pull-downs or pull-ups; some sort of rowing motion; and then some tricep dips and bicep curls for those smaller muscles. There are examples of these types of exercises in Chapter 9 and on the *Fit Moms for Life* DVDs.

Last, but not least, include core exercises. We'll talk about core more specifically later in this chapter. When working

> " When you're doing your workout, you really should push yourself as much as possible. You're there for 45 minutes. Make it count! Use the heaviest weights you possibly can while keeping good form. Focus on a mental image of what you are trying to achieve during that time."
>
> – Kelly

your core, focus on the deep core first—the bigger muscles—and then work the outer core.

As you put together your workouts, keep in mind that you don't need more than one or two different exercises per body part. There are different ways to approach the sets and reps that you do, and it's important to mix that up. For example, in the *Fit Moms for Life* DVD series, the first couple of DVDs have you doing two to three sets, with 10 to 15 reps, and you're probably not using really heavy weights because your body is just getting used to this kind of exercise. But then as the DVDs progress, some workouts have you doing four sets of six reps. When there are fewer reps, it means you're using heavier weights. Then we'll go back to higher reps with lower weights for another workout. It's really important to work all the different muscles at different levels, and to keep your body guessing what's coming next.

Finally, to keep your exercise time to a minimum and to keep your heart rate up, don't rest too long between sets of an exercise. You can work through a circuit, where you go through all the exercises you're going to do once and then go back through for a second set of everything. Another option is to do a pair of exercises back-to-back, work through all your sets with those two, and move on to the next pair. (For example, you might do a set of dead lifts and a set of push-ups, and then do your second set of each of those before you move on to different exercises.)

> I used to lift light weights, lots of reps, on my lunch hour. And looking back I just think that was so much time wasted. I never saw the results that I have now."
>
> – Amber

Using Challenging Weights

I hope I've convinced you by now that strength training is going to help you get into the best shape of your life. But it's not just about doing any kind of strength training. I believe this transformation is going to take place only when you use challenging weights.

Now, of course, what qualifies as "challenging" will depend on your current strength and what exercise you're doing. The simple guideline to go by is that you want to use a weight that's very difficult for the exercise you're doing for as many reps as you are trying to do.

Let's say I'm prescribing 12 reps for a shoulder press. Many women would pick 5-pound weights, and they would do the 12 reps with little to no difficulty. They probably could do 20 to 25 reps before it got really difficult. On the other hand, if they heard me saying they needed to use challenging weights, they might go a little overboard, pick up the 25-pounders right off the bat, and find that they could only do one to three reps. Clearly, that would be too heavy for the exercise and their current strength level. You want to choose a weight that allows you to keep good

> It's fun to feel like what I have lifted over my head or on my shoulders is bigger than I am, or at least weighs almost as much as I do!"
>
> – Sarah

form, but one you find very difficult to lift by the 12th rep. (For the record, I'd rather see you try the 25-pound weights, realize it's too hard, and go down to 20- or 15-pounders, than do the 12 reps with 5-pound weights and say, "Oh, that was easy.")

Note that as you're getting started, I'm not encouraging you to dive in with the most challenging weights you can find. The first couple of weeks, your body is adjusting and you are figuring out your form and what you can handle, so I wouldn't push the heavy weights. Your muscles, tendons, and ligaments need to get stronger to get your whole body ready for more intense strength training, and that can take up to a month. But even during that first month, don't use the really, really light weights. Even if you haven't done strength training before, you will probably be able to handle at least 10-pound weights for most upper-body exercises (except things like lateral

> *I was definitely skeptical about hefting around those heavy weights, especially because I've always been on the large end of the spectrum for a female. I'm like, 'Am I going to get all buffed up and turn into a thick-necked woman named Gunther?' That never happened, and I don't worry about it at all anymore. It can't happen."*
> — Trish

raises, where you'd probably want to start with 5-pounders), and 15- to 20-pound weights for lower-body exercises. In Chapter 9 you'll see the recommended weights to start with for each exercise.

If you use my *Fit Moms for Life* DVDs, you'll be watching women who have undergone amazing transformations, who have worked super hard, and who are now very strong and lean. I don't necessarily want you to compete with them, but I chose them because I wanted you to see what is possible. In some of the DVDs, you'll see my clients lifting 50-pound dumbbells. I don't expect you to go out and buy 50-pounders or to be able to lift those right away. None of my clients could lift those when they started, either, and they probably wouldn't have believed me if I'd told them that someday, they'd be starring in a fitness DVD and lifting 50-pound dumbbells. I bet you're capable of more than you think. I also like to show these lean, toned women lifting heavy weights to reassure you that you're not going to bulk up as you use the heavier weights.

Core Training

While we're talking about strength training, I think it's really important to discuss core training. Strengthening the core was my first passion—even back when I was a scrawny teenager, I worked hard to develop and maintain a six-pack. It's an area where I have a lot of expertise, and there are so many misunderstandings out there about how to get a flat stomach and how to exercise these critical muscles.

> *My core is incredibly tight and pulled in, and I don't have the back problems that I used to have. And my stomach is relatively flat all the time."*
> — Abby

First, let's get the myth out of the way: Just doing hundreds of ab exercises is not going to get you a flat stomach. What you really need to do first is get rid of the fat on the whole body. You can have the strongest core muscles in the world, but with a layer of fat over them, no one's ever going to see them and your stomach is never going to be flat. That's why core exercise needs to be part of a larger program that includes eating right and exercising your whole body. Crunches in particular—which many people think are the key to a flat stomach—are not effective from a fat-burning perspective because they exercise a pretty small muscle group.

The core muscles are very important for everyday activities and especially for the health of your back. The Mayo Clinic says that 80 percent of people have lower-back issues at some point in their lives. Most of those people could be either helped or cured by doing core exercises and properly training those muscles. I've seen this with many of my clients. Some people come to me barely able to lift a pencil without risking lower-back pain. Once they start doing proper core training, they are able to do more and more—in life and in the gym. I have some guys who have gone from not being able to work out at all to lifting 200 pounds in just a year or two.

> ### Understanding the Anatomy
> A lot of muscles make up what we call the core. The transverse abdominal muscles are your deep core. They run parallel to the ground, cinching in your stomach and keeping your spine and abdominal area tight. The internal and external oblique muscles wrap around the sides of your abdomen; they help you twist side to side and bend sideways. The rectus abdominis (your six-pack or eight-pack) is the outer abs, which extend down below your belly button. Those are the crunching muscles. Then you have the erector spinae muscles in your lower back. There are other muscles in the core, but those are the main ones, and you need to train all of them to have a strong core.

Most people go about core exercises the wrong way. They start from the outside first, so they do the crunches and work on the outer abs, the least important muscle for core strength. I've met so many moms who thought crunches were going to be their best friend to get their stomach back after having a baby. But working the outer abs right after pregnancy can actually make your stomach look worse! If your deep core muscles aren't strong, then when you do a crunch, you're going to see your abdomen peak. Maybe it's happened to you: You crunch up, and your abs stick up. That's a result of not engaging the deep core. After pregnancy, you need to recover your deep core

> *In a big snowstorm recently, I was out shoveling and I could feel my core engaging and working to lift the heavy snow. It just makes everything in life so much easier."*
> – Karen E.

strength before you start doing too many crunches. (See Appendix A on "Fitness for New Moms and Moms-to-Be" for more advice about recovering from pregnancy and childbirth.)

The key to any exercise program is variety, so there's no one best exercise. You should try to hit all the major core muscles each time you work your core. My *Got Core* DVD program includes eight 15-minute workouts you can do on a stability ball. They're great, challenging, quick workouts that hit the core from all different angles. Below, I'll go through which exercises work each of the major muscle groups in the core—many of these are described in the sample workout in Chapter 9. If you have chronic lower back pain, I recommend getting the *Got Core* DVDs, but also picking up a copy of the best-selling book, *The 7-Day Back Pain Cure: How Thousands of People Got Relief Without Doctors, Drugs, or Surgery*, by my friend Jesse Cannone.

Transverse abdominals. My recommendation is to work the deep core first and the most. There are a lot of terrific exercises for this. The first one is planks. Planks are very popular, but I don't think enough people do them, and those who do tend to put them toward the end of the workout as an afterthought. I'd recommend that you start out holding a front plank for 30 seconds to a minute. (You can hold it for longer if you like, but if you go longer than two to three minutes, I'm not sure you're getting any added benefits. Rather than holding it longer and longer, increase the difficulty by lifting one leg or putting either your forearms or your toes on a stability ball.) I also recommend you do side planks, holding them for 30 seconds to a minute on each side. Those are really going to work those deep core muscles.

My other recommendation for strengthening your deep core muscles is called the vacuum exercise. This is basically an exercise where you draw in your abdominal muscles and hold your breath for 10 seconds. (See the full description and picture on page 128.) This is awesome for anyone, but especially for newer moms who haven't regained the strength in their deep core muscles. You can actually trim two to four inches off your waist within a couple of months by doing this exercise on a daily basis. It doesn't burn away the fat around your waist—it just trains your body to keep your abdomen pulled in. You can't really overtrain on this one, and it's something you can do throughout the day. I'd recommend doing 10 to 15 vacuums each day. You can do it while you're cooking, driving, lying in bed, watching TV—there's really no excuse not to do it. Over time, your body is going to get used to that feeling, and it's just going to naturally be drawn in as those muscles are engaged more often. That's not only going to help prevent or decrease lower-back injuries and pain, but it's also going to make your waist appear a lot smaller.

Obliques. To strengthen your obliques, you can do any sort of twisting exercise. I like the Russian twist, where you balance on your tailbone and twist back and forth. You can hold a weight and touch it to the ground on either side of you, or just touch the ground with your hands. I also recommend doing some sort of oblique crunch. For example, you can lie with one hip on a stability ball, hands at your ears, and your feet up against a wall. Drape your body over the stability ball, and then bend at your side to bring your body into a straight line. Repeat 10 to 15 times, then switch to the other side. Side planks are also good for the obliques.

Lower back. Back extension exercises are great for strengthening the lower back, as are "swimmers." You want to extend the back and lift the chest up, whether you're on the floor or on a stability ball.

Lower abdominal area. Most people are self-conscious about their lower abs, right below the belly button, especially moms. Even for me, as a guy, that's where I find I put on fat. As I've said before, losing body fat through total-body exercise and proper nutrition is what you really need to do. But there are a few exercises you can do that will help tone and tighten that area. You want to do some sort of leg-raise motion. I like one called the foot-to-hand transfer with a ball. Lie down on your back with a stability ball in your hands above your head. Transfer the ball from your hands to your feet, crunching up as your hands and feet are above your stomach, and then lower the ball to the ground between your feet. And then back to the hands, and so on. Another option is to do an exercise where you're lying down with your legs straight up in the air. Lift

> " My waistline was the part of my body that bothered me the most after having babies—and the one I found hardest to get back. But with MamaTone, I've lost at least six inches around my waist. And it isn't just the number of inches around, but what my stomach looks like. There may still be a teeny bit of something there that I don't like to look at, but I went on a trip awhile ago and wore a bikini. And for the first time in a long time, I didn't feel self-conscious about my stomach."
> – Sarah

your butt off the ground a bit—just a couple of inches. It's a small motion. It's like a crunch where you're lifting with your lower abs instead of your upper abs. The vacuums I described before are also going to help pull in your lower abs.

Outer abs. Last—and I think least important—are the outer abs, and the crunching exercises most people do. When you do crunches, try to really engage the deep core so that you're drawing in your belly button toward your spine. Focus on controlling your movement and going slowly, and you won't need to go above 15 to 20 reps. People often brag that they do 200 crunches a day. Well, crunches aren't the greatest exercise to spend all your time on, and doing that many reps isn't the greatest either. It's probably a sign that you're just using momentum and not really focusing on the muscles you're working. Hold a weight above you for resistance if you need to and make it hard for yourself, so that you're fatigued by 15 or 20 reps.

The *Got Core* DVD set includes eight short workouts that work all of these muscles. You can also get my Flat Stomach app for the iPhone (just search for "flat stomach workout" on iTunes), which allows you to put together a workout, choosing the exercises you want to do for the amount of time you have.

Working Up to a Pull-Up

So many women are intimidated by the thought of doing a pull-up. And in fact, very few women can do one—probably fewer than one in 1,000. So it's pretty rare, but I have at least 50 female clients that can do one pull-up, and many of them can do several. With the new focus on lean strength in women, I think we will see a lot more women doing pull-ups.

If you can't do a pull-up today, there are a lot of different ways to work up to doing one. If you're in a gym, they might have an assisted pull-up machine that lifts some of your body weight for you. The heavier you put the stack, the easier it gets. That's a nice way to go about it. As you get stronger and lose weight, you will need less and less assistance, and eventually you'll be able to lift your body weight without any help. You can also try it with different grips. For a true pull-up, your palms are facing away from you. If your palms are facing in, that's a chin-up, which is a bit easier.

Another machine to use at the gym is a lat pull-down machine. With that one, you're pulling down the weight using the same muscles you use for a pull-up, and you can gradually build up the amount you're able to pull down.

You don't have to be at the gym to work on this, though. Let's say you spend a lot of time at the playground. Use the monkey bars to strengthen your muscles and show off for the neighborhood kids. Hold two bars about shoulder-width apart, and jump up so that your chin is up by the bars (or as far up as you can get). Then slowly lower yourself. That's called a negative, and I'd say it's even more effective at building strength than the pulling-up motion itself. Your biceps and back have to work hard to achieve that slow lowering of the body.

Some other ways to build up to doing a pull-up would be to have a chair underneath you or a partner holding your legs, so that they can lift up or you can kind of push up off your legs to remove some of the weight, and then lower yourself. You can also practice isolation, where you jump up halfway and hold yourself there for five to 10 seconds with your elbows at a 90-degree angle, and then lower yourself. Finally, the biggest thing you can do to improve your pull-ups is to lose weight if you're overweight. It's just really difficult for a woman to develop upper-body muscles strong enough to lift higher amounts of weight. The closer you can get to your ideal weight, the easier a pull-up will be.

Soreness After Strength Training

People who are new to strength training, or who haven't done it in a long time, get caught off guard by how sore they are the next day. There's a 48- to 72-hour period after strength training when you will definitely be sore. It's called delayed onset muscle soreness, but no one really knows exactly why it happens. When you first start my

> *"I remember being so sore for a couple of days after my first class and thinking, 'This is what I need.'"*
>
> – Liz

program, you might experience the "hit by a bus" syndrome and have a hard time moving around for two to three days. I promise you that after a week or two of that, you will stop having that extreme soreness and will just be able to feel which muscles you really challenged. Most of my clients get to a point where they miss that soreness if they don't work out; or if they don't hurt at least a little bit the next day after a workout, they feel like they got ripped off. Hopefully, you'll get to that point, too.

In the meantime, there are three things you can do to help with the soreness. One is to keep moving. Stay active. The more you sit around and complain about how sore you are, the worse it's going to get. Do some body-weight squats, do some lunges. If your arms and chest are sore, move them around and keep them limber. Another thing you can do is to take an Epsom salt bath, which can help draw toxins out of the muscles and keep things warm. The final thing is to drink water. When you're well hydrated, your body will be able to flush out the lactic acid that builds up from strength training. Hang in there—it will get better if you can get past those first two weeks.

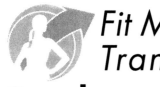

Fit Moms for Life Transformation

Sarah

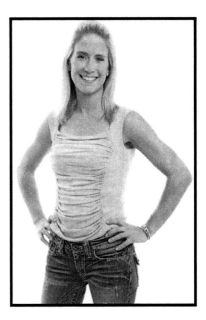

My client and friend Sarah is a TV news anchor. What she's gone through in the past two years would have convinced many people to put fitness on the back burner, but she stayed consistent with her exercise and is one of the strongest women I know at 113 pounds.

Sarah's story: "Most of my life, I've been petite, around 115 pounds, and luckily able to stay that way. I was a dancer growing up and got into running, and that worked for me for many years. But after my second baby, it just didn't seem to be doing it anymore. When I met Dustin, my youngest was six months old and I was about 138 pounds. Some of that was still post-pregnancy weight, but it wasn't coming off fast enough with running and doing crunches at home.

Sarah, 35, mother of two. 5'3", 113 pounds. Sarah got back to her high school and college weight after having two kids, including losing six inches off her waist.

"Two years ago, I was diagnosed with epilepsy. It was quite a mystery to doctors. About six months ago they found a tumor in my brain that was causing the seizures, and I had surgery to remove it. Luckily, it was not cancerous and I'm about as healthy as a person could be after going through that. So I feel very blessed. But I also went through a divorce, which was final about a year ago. I can count on one hand the things that helped me survive the divorce, a disease that I didn't understand, two small children, and a job that entailed waking up at 3 a.m.—and I honestly believe Dustin's program was among them. I somehow knew that if I kept that workout routine going, it would help me survive."

Sarah's exercise tips: "Don't make excuses not to work out. It's really easy to find a reason you're too busy or too tired. There's always something life throws at us that adds stress and makes us 'too busy.' But I showed up to MamaTone twice a week throughout everything else that was happening because it made a difference for me. So I think you can make it happen with whatever's going on in your life."

Read more of Sarah's story at *fitmomsforlife.com/sarah.*

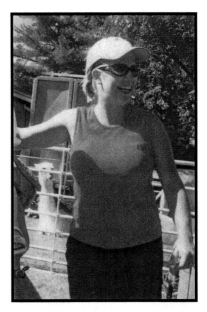

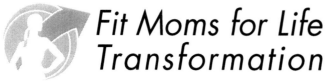

Fit Moms for Life Transformation

Donna

Donna is a great example of a woman in her forties who has been able to achieve great results through my program.

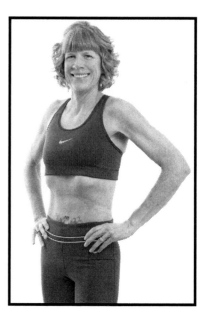

Donna's story: "Before I heard about Dustin's program, I had lost 50 pounds from my highest weight ever, and was down to a size 6, mostly by changing the way I ate in some of the same ways that Dustin recommends. With the *Fit Moms for Life* DVDs, I lost an additional 15 pounds and am now a size 2.

"I thought I was in fairly good shape when I started the program, but I had hardly ever done push-ups on my toes. I could do maybe three, and they were really bad. Now I can do 20 like a piece of cake. I was skeptical about whether I could lift the heavy weights at my age, but I've worked my way up to 30-pound dumbbells! I've been amazed what I can do when I put my mind to it.

"Before doing Dustin's program, I had premenopausal symptoms. I was having night sweats and foggy brain, and was feeling really crappy. My doctor suggested I take antidepressants. Instead, I started Dustin's program. I am pretty much symptom-free now. I feel completely different."

Donna's current goals: "I'm hoping to be the most ripped 50-year-old I know!"

Donna's nutrition tips: "The biggest thing for me is the four to five small meals a day, because then you're never hungry. As soon as you start to feel hungry, you eat something little. And then you're good until you eat again."

Donna's advice to you: "It's tough, but you can do it. Don't tell yourself you can't. Just try it and keep going, and you will get the results you want. And you'll be happier and feel great, too."

Read more of Donna's story at *fitmomsforlife.com/donna*.

Donna, 48.
5'8", 125 pounds.
Donna went from a size 18 to a size 2 by changing her eating habits and working out with the Fit Moms for Life DVDs in her home.

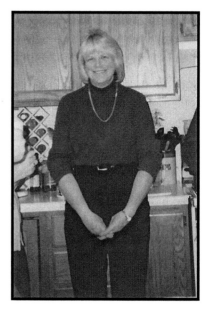

The New Rules of Cardio

You've probably caught on by now that I'm never going to recommend you spend hours a day on the treadmill or the elliptical machine. I actually think training for a marathon is a terrible strategy for getting in shape or losing weight. (I know some people love to run and I can see the value of setting a challenging goal and the thrill of achieving it—but that doesn't mean it's going to help you lose weight!) If you hate running or you hate cardio, you've come to the right place. I will never prescribe much of it. But I will describe how you can use short bursts of intense cardiovascular exercise to accelerate your weight loss and help you get into the best shape of your life.

Why Cardio Makes People Fat

The idea that steady-state, long-duration cardio exercise is the best way or the only way to burn fat is pretty pervasive, so I want to start by telling you why I believe that kind of cardio actually makes people fat. The idea of the "fat-burning zone" started in the 1980s or 1990s when researchers looked at differing levels of exercise intensity and the percentage of fat and carbs burned. This is a little confusing, but stay with me and I'll explain it.

When you're doing lower-intensity exercise such as walking, you burn a very high percentage of fat relative to carbs. If you're doing something like intense strength training or sprinting, for example, you're going to be burning mostly carbs, so the percentage of fat being burned is lower. That's why low-intensity cardio was considered the "fat-burning zone"—but there are a couple problems with that logic.

First of all, the lower your intensity, the smaller your overall calorie burn. So even if the percentage of fat being burned is high, the amount of fat burned is still going to be pretty low. With higher intensity, you're burning more calories overall, so you're burning more fat calories even though they make up a smaller percentage of the calories being used.

The other issue is the after-burn effect, which I described in Chapter 7. The less intense exercise you do, the quicker your metabolism goes back to its normal level. So the higher the intensity of your workout, the longer your metabolism will be raised afterward. That adds up to a lot more fat calories burned in the long run.

Another negative aspect of running or other steady-state cardio is that it eats away muscle. Especially when it's coupled with a low-calorie diet, relying on steady-state cardio can throw people into a cycle in which their metabolism gets lower and lower and they have to keep increasing their cardio or decreasing their calories to maintain their weight loss.

Over the years, our bodies have evolved to be very good at survival. If you're training for a marathon and you're consistently putting a lot of miles on each week, your body knows it needs a significant amount of energy to do that. And your body actually knows what researchers took awhile to figure out—that it needs to burn fat to sustain that lower-intensity exercise. So, once you've been doing that kind of training for a while, your body starts to say, "I don't necessarily need to burn through all these carbs right now. I need to store some as fat to use during long runs." Your body actually starts to store more fat in case it needs it for running.

> *You need the cardio, the strength training, and the core. You cannot have just one of those things. You need all of those components to really be fit. For me, it's not just about losing weight, but having a body that is strong and healthy. And just doing cardio is not going to do that."*
>
> – Crystal

The other issue when people spend a lot of time on cardio is that they start to eat more. Part of it may be a physical increase in appetite—the research on that is inconclusive, but I've seen it with many of my clients, and I believe a lot of running and a lot of cardio really does increase your appetite more than strength training does. But there's also the mentality that goes along with it. You're exercising so long that you feel it justifies eating anything you want. "Man, I just did two hours of exercise. I can eat this pizza now." Well, in your two hours of exercise you might have burned 1,000 calories, if it was a good workout. Then you could easily eat three pieces of pizza, and that's 1,000 calories right there. And it's probably not where you stop. You'd likely have dessert, or a beer, or one more slice. You end up consuming more calories than you actually burned.

While we're on the topic of running, there's another point I'd like to make: People who are new to exercise or who haven't exercised in a long time often go out and try to run when they decide it's time to get in shape. The thing is, running in itself is a very athletic activity. It requires a lot of strength, coordination, and flexibility. You've got to be healthy to do it. Unfortunately, we have a lot of unhealthy, unfit people running to try to get in shape—and I think that's why so many people hate exercise, because they're doing something their body is not ready for. Not to mention that they're risking injury when they go from not exercising at all to running. One study showed that about 65 percent of runners experience at least one injury per year.[1] Another showed even higher injury rates, as high as 90 percent, among those training for a marathon.[2]

The good news for people who do enjoy running is that you can decrease the likelihood of injuring yourself while running if you add more variety to your training. Replace one or two runs per week with strength training. You'll strengthen your muscles and your core and put less strain on your joints. My client Karen, an accomplished runner and running coach, said, "Running healthy has been a big benefit of strength training—I've had a lot fewer injuries, no more pains, no more overuse injuries."

> " Every time I wanted to get in shape, I'd run. Well, when you haven't run in forever, you know, suddenly taking up long-distance running doesn't work. I'd injure myself or get shin splints or something and I'd give up."
>
> – Katy

Shift Your Focus to Intensity

Rather than spend hours burning a low number of calories, we need to redirect our focus to more intense exercise that will raise the heart rate, burn a lot of calories, and generate a good after-burn. This shift started in the late 1990s, when fitness professionals started talking about interval training. The idea was that instead of, say, running for an hour straight at the same intensity, we should start to mix it up. For one minute we'd run at 60 percent of our max, the next minute was at 70 percent, the next was at 80 percent, and then we brought it down to 50 percent again and cycled through that, increasing the intensity and decreasing it again. People saw better results from that than they had from steady-state cardio. They saw their times go down on runs. They became better at using oxygen. It was really an awesome development.

The burst training I'm recommending is the next step in that direction. Research in the last five years has shown that training more like a sprinter is even more effective. I bet you've never seen a fat sprinter, and they never run for more than 30 seconds. Burst training is the new gold standard for weight loss.

For busy moms, the beauty of burst training is that instead of doing an hour of cardio, you only have to do about 15 minutes. Plus, it's going to be more effective because you're burning more calories and more fat, and you're raising your metabolism for a longer period with the more intense workout. So as you go on with the rest of your day—showering, taking the kids to school, going to work—your metabolism is still elevated and burning extra calories.

1 Lysholm, J., and J. Wiklander. "Injuries in Runners." American Journal of Sports Medicine 15.2 (1987): 168-71.
2 Satterthwaite, P., et al. "Incidence of Injuries and Other Health Problems in the Auckland Citibank Marathon, 1993." British Journal of Sports Medicine 30.44 (1996): 324-26.

How to Incorporate Burst Training

There are a lot of ways to go about it, but the basic idea is that you're going to work at a very high intensity for somewhere between 10 seconds and a minute. (If you go longer than a minute, it's really more of an interval training program.) So you might do something for 30 seconds as hard as you can. Whether it's running, swimming, climbing stairs, or doing jumping jacks, you're doing it as intensely as possible. You could even lie on the ground and throw a tantrum like your kid. The point is to work so hard that after 30 seconds, you've nearly reached your maximum heart rate. You want to be at a level of exertion around a nine or 10 on a scale of 10.

After 30 seconds, you stop doing whatever you're doing and let your body recover. (If you're running or climbing, you might slow down to a walk or just stand for a while to recover. On a treadmill, you can straddle the treadmill during your rest period, so that you don't have to keep lowering and raising the speed.) Your rest

> **"** *The burst cardio is really, really hard, but short. I enjoy the challenge."*
> – Sarah

period might be as long as four times the work period—so in this example, where you worked for 30 seconds, you'd rest for two minutes. As you get fitter, you can cut that down to more like a 3:1, 2:1, or even 1:1 ratio of resting to working. After the rest period, you do another 30 seconds of very hard work, and then you rest again, and you keep alternating like that. See the table on this page for some sample programs to work through. Each program indicates how many seconds you'll be "on" and how many you'll be "off" for the duration of your workout. Move up through the programs as you increase your cardiovascular endurance over time.

Burst Training Programs

Program	Seconds on	Seconds off
1	60	180
2	30	120
3	15	45
4	60	120
5	30	60
6	15	30
7	60	60
8	30	30
9	15	15

You'll need a few minutes to warm up (using a dynamic warm-up, as illustrated in Chapter 9) and maybe a couple of less-intense intervals to get started. Then you'll want to do five to 12 intervals at high intensity, depending on the length of them and your fitness level. With a two-minute cooldown at the end, the whole workout will last 10 to 20 minutes. (If you're adding burst training to the end of a strength training workout, you can do just five to 10 minutes—your body is already warmed up and ready to go.) There's no reason you couldn't do burst training three, four, even five times a week in addition to your strength training. At a minimum, you want to do it twice a week.

You'll be amazed at what you can do. Obviously, it's super-hard work. You sweat a lot. I guess you could say it's a lot more uncomfortable than steady-state cardio, but it's more time-efficient and more effective—and it keeps it interesting, too. The time flies by when you're changing up the pace like that.

Of course, you need to take some precautions with burst training. You have to be careful about the impact on your joints from that intense activity, even though it's only for a short time. If you're running or doing jump squats or another high-impact exercise, you want to be careful about how often you do it. Maybe mix it up with swimming or another lower-impact burst activity some days. You also need to pay attention to your body. I want you to push yourself and get close to your maximum heart rate—but you need to know your limit, and stop if it's too much. If you feel nauseated or light-headed, or really can't catch your breath after an interval, slow down or stop. Gradually increase what you can do as you learn how much you can push yourself.

Burst Training Activities

There are so many different ways to get your heart rate up, in a gym, in your house, or in the great outdoors. Here are a few ideas that work well for short bursts of intensity:

- Running
- Swimming*
- Climbing stairs (If you're in a tall building, take the elevator down for your rest period, to reduce the impact on your knees.)
- Sledding (Run up, sled down!)
- Biking*
- Burpees
- Jumping jacks
- Lying on the ground and throwing a tantrum*
- Speed walking uphill*

*Lower-impact activities for people with knee problems.

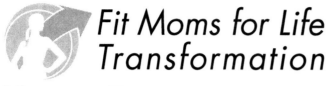

Fit Moms for Life Transformation

Karen E.

Karen had always been a runner, but since she started doing the *Fit Moms for Life* DVDs, she has converted to strength training! She is now a certified personal trainer and one of my boot camp instructors.

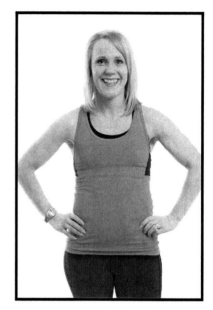

Karen's story: "Running always fit well with my lifestyle. I could push my kids in a stroller. I used to travel a lot for work, and I could run anywhere on the road. I coached high school track and ran races from 5Ks to a marathon. But after my third child, I just wasn't getting back into the kind of shape I wanted to be in. I started doing *Fit Moms for Life* in my basement in June. I couldn't believe the results I was seeing by the end of the summer. I was much stronger. I could see definition in my arms. I no longer had lower-back pain. And I was running faster and stronger than I ever had, which was amazing to me. After two months of doing *FMFL*—and a lot less running than I used to do—I ran a 5K. I took five minutes off from my time a year earlier. My pace was just under seven minutes a mile, which is fast. I also dropped about 15 pounds in weight. Everything just got smaller and tighter.

Karen E., 39, mother of three. 5'2", 115 pounds. Karen used the Fit Moms for Life DVDs to lose 15 pounds, tone up, and improve her running times.

"I love that I am a positive role model for my three girls. They can do anything that they want to do. I'm teaching them from a young age that fitness is an important part of their lives and women can be strong. We don't have to wait for Dad to open that jar—we can open it ourselves!"

Karen's nutrition tips: "As crazy as it sounds, make a spreadsheet with your meal plan for the week. It works! When you're crunched on time, anyone in the house can look at the spreadsheet and chip in to help."

Karen's advice to you: "If you aren't in shape or you've never tried strength training, just jump in and try it. Yes, the first couple of weeks will be hard. You'll have muscle soreness, but it is so worth it to treat yourself to that 45 minutes of giving your body what it needs to be strong and healthy for the future."

Read more of Karen's story at *fitmomsforlife.com/karene.*

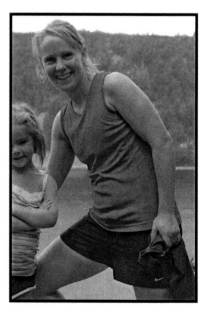

Fit Moms for Life Transformation

Lynn

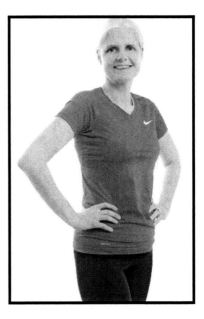

Lynn has quietly transformed her body over the past year with a soft determination that I love.

Lynn's story: "I started this journey three years ago, after the birth of my second child, at my heaviest weight ever, 190 pounds. I started by making small changes. I made better food choices and committed to exercising a few times a week. As the weight started to come off, I felt more comfortable and confident and decided to join a running group. My weight went down to 150 pounds, but then back up to 165, and I became frustrated. I decided to try Dustin's program. I've been going to boot camp three times a week for a little over a year now, and I am down to 130 pounds. For the majority of my life, I have not been overweight, so I feel as though I have myself back now. I feel more confident and I have more energy for my life.

Lynn, 36, mother of two. 5'5", 130 pounds. Lynn dropped 60 pounds and seven dress sizes—from a 22 to an 8—through my boot camps.

"One of the biggest things I have gained is a feeling of control. Being overweight made me feel out of control and overwhelmed. Now I feel more in control and confident. When you push through an extra mile of running or that last repetition of weights, it translates to the rest of your life. I feel better prepared to manage everyday life stresses like when one of my boys has a tantrum or my plans get turned upside down."

Lynn's current goals: "My goal is to keep this weight off and not fall into my pattern of dropping my good habits once I've accomplished a goal. I plan to lose five more pounds so I have a little wiggle room. Plus, I've just signed up to train for my first half marathon!"

Lynn's exercise tips: "Even if it's not your best day, if you just keep working, you're going to get to your goal. Sometimes just the fact that you're there is what's important; you're not sitting on the couch. Some days are great, some days are not so great, but you've just got to keep getting out there and doing it. Slow and steady is the name of the game."

Read more of Lynn's story at *fitmomsforlife.com/lynn.*

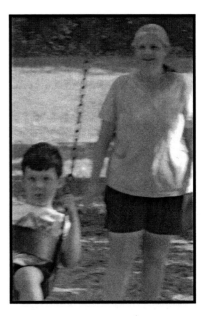

Putting Together an Exercise Routine

I've given you a lot of information about strength training and burst training. Now I want to help you find a routine that will allow you to incorporate these kinds of exercise into your life and share a sample workout you can use to get started.

Working Out at Home: Home Exercise Equipment

Home workouts are the right choice for many people. If you're short on time or you can't find a gym that meets your childcare needs, or you're just the type of person who prefers to work out alone, working out at home is a great solution. You will need some equipment to do it right, though.

First, of course, you'll need some **dumbbells**. I'd say most women starting out should have a set of 8-pound or 10-pound dumbbells, and then sets of 15s, 20s, and maybe 25s. If you're really weak, you could also get 5-pounders, but people tend to fall back on those as a crutch, so I don't recommend having them in the house. (There are only a few exercises where I would recommend using 5-pound weights, like lateral raises. Eight-pounders work for that too, though.) As you get stronger, you can keep adding heavier ones to your collection. Some of my clients think of this like collecting shoes or purses. I've had a lot of people ask me whether the variable-resistance dumbbells are worthwhile. Those are the ones where you turn a knob or take a pin out to change the weight. I think I've tried every brand out there, and I find them really hard to work with. They're not very comfortable, and they're not as durable as regular dumbbells. So while they seem like a good idea, I'd stick with the old-fashioned kind.

Dumbbells can be expensive. Usually, you're looking at about $1 per pound. If you keep an eye on

Craigslist in your area, you might see some come up for sale, but it's pretty rare. You can also check garage sales and used exercise equipment stores, or just put out the word to your friends and family that you're looking for dumbbells—a lot of people have some in the basement that they never use, so maybe you could get lucky.

The next thing I highly recommend is a **stability ball** (or an ab ball, or a Swiss ball—there are a lot of different names for it). When you go to buy one, you'll see there are different sizes, too. I recommend most people get a 55-centimeter ball. A quality ball will cost you about $20—don't go for the cheapest one you can find, because the ones made from thinner material will start to lose their shape as you sit on them.

Another thing you'll need for some exercises is something you can use as a **bench or step**. It's got to be something really solid, like a piano bench or a flat, sturdy chair. For some exercises, you can use the second step on a stairwell. You're looking for something that's 18 to 24 inches high that can hold your weight for step-up exercises and tricep dip exercises.

Then there are a couple of optional things. If you're working out on a wood floor, you might want to have a **yoga mat** to make things a little softer when you're lying down. Some people like to use **workout gloves** so they don't get calluses from the weights.

If you only need a stability ball and a couple of dumbbells, you could get set up to do my program at home with an initial expense of less than $50. (Depending on the weights you use and what else you need for your situation, you could spend a lot more than that, but that would be enough to get started.) It shouldn't take much space in your house, either. You can put all of it in a corner somewhere. The ball will take up a little bit of space, but you can actually use it to sit on while you watch TV or use the computer. And I bet your kids will want to play with it all the time, too.

Working Out at a Gym: What to Look For

If working out at home isn't for you, a gym might be the best option. They will have all the equipment I recommend and more. Just make sure before signing a gym membership that it's something you're going to use. Make sure it fits your needs. If you need childcare, is it included with your membership? Are there specific classes you want to attend? Is the gym too crowded during the times you are looking to go? The Y is a good low-cost option in most communities, with lots of activities for children and families, too.

Gyms can also be a great place to meet others, so join a gym if you're looking for workout buddies or the extra motivation of being around other people who are working hard.

Your Exercise Routine

I recommend you strength train your whole body three days every week, and do burst training at least two or three days a week. Let's look at different ways to put together those workouts and what will be most effective in terms of time and calorie-burning. There are two different options I recommend, and you can choose the one that works best with your preferences and schedule. You can commit roughly an hour a day for three or four days a week, or about 30 minutes for five or six days a week. I believe that shorter workouts more days of the week are more effective, but of course, that doesn't work for everyone's schedule. You can still get great results with hour-long workouts three to four days a week.

Hour-long exercise, three to four days per week. You want to include strength training on three of your exercise days, working both your upper and lower body each time. You need to let your muscles rest and recover, so I recommend you exercise every other day and try not to do the strength training on two consecutive days.

I prefer to start with a dynamic workout for a few minutes (see page 121 for more information) and then go into 30 minutes of strength training—maybe 45 minutes, tops, but 30 should be enough. Then do 10 to 15 minutes of burst training and five to 10 minutes of core work before you stretch. That's the structure my *Fit Moms for Life* DVDs follow, and it takes about an hour to do a whole DVD. I don't like to work out more than an hour. I think with anything beyond that, you get diminishing returns.

There has been substantial research about whether you should do your cardio before or after your strength training. More of the research supports doing the cardio afterward as the way to burn more fat. I really think of it more in terms of the energy you have available for the different parts of your workout. When you do your cardio first, you're so tired that you don't have the energy to push yourself in the strength training portion.

When you're doing this kind of workout three days a week, you might want to throw in a little extra training on one of your off days. That's when I'd recommend going for a longer bike ride or a swim or a run. Taking a yoga, Pilates, Zumba, or spinning class is a great option, too. Just choose something you enjoy doing.

Shorter exercise five to six days per week. If you're going to exercise five to six days a week, there are a couple different ways you can structure your workouts. The first is to alternate lower-body and upper-body workouts for a shorter strength training portion. That way, your lower-body muscles are recovering the day you're working your upper body, and vice versa. That might take about 20 minutes, and then you can alternate whether you use the remaining time for burst training or core work. (Of course, you need to warm up before your workout and stretch afterward, no matter how you structure it.)

The other way to set up shorter, more frequent workouts is to do 30 minutes of full-body strength training one day and do core work and burst training for about 30 minutes the next. This is very easy to do with the *Fit Moms for Life* DVDs, because the portions are already the right lengths and the full-body workout is already put together for you. You could even use my *Got Core* workout to add some variety and new challenges for your core work. If you want to do something extra or different like yoga, that's fine. Just make sure you get three days' worth of strength training in for both upper and lower body.

Warming Up

In the past, warming up to exercise meant holding a static stretch. You probably did this at the beginning of gym class when you were a kid. You'd be doing the hurdler stretch, where you're sitting on the ground with your legs in front of you and reaching your hands for your toes, trying to stretch your lower back and hamstrings. I still see people doing this all the time. Recently, a lot of large studies have shown that this type of stretching, especially if you do it when your muscles are still cold, either decreases performance and increases the risk of injury, or does not do anything at all.

What I recommend is called a dynamic warm-up. The idea is to prepare your body for the movements that will occur in your workout. So if you're going to be running, start off with a walk, pick it up to a fast walk, and then go to a slow jog.

To prepare for a strength training workout, your warm-up needs to involve all the muscles you will work. I like to do movements similar to the exercises coming up, but with no weight. Squats, lunges, arm circles, pushing, and rowing motions are all good. You're not using any weights, just working the motion. As you get more warmed up, you can make it more intense, adding in some jumps and other things that will start to get your heart going. The sample workout in this chapter includes a dynamic warm-up you can use.

A dynamic warm-up can last anywhere from three to 10 minutes. You don't want to be out of breath from your warm-up, but you might be starting to break a sweat and you should feel your heart beating a bit faster. As you age, it might take you a little bit longer to warm up, so give yourself the time you need to feel ready for your workout.

Sample Workout

The following workout is the same as you'll find on the first *Fit Moms for Life* DVD—and I even got the star of that DVD, Jody, to model for these photos. Start doing this workout on your own at home, and if you like it, go to my website and sign up to get a year's worth of workouts just like it. Each DVD provides you with a challenging workout, getting harder as you go through the year and get stronger. Each one features a mom, like Jody and the other women you've met throughout this book, who has made impressive gains in her fitness through my program. You can learn more at *fitmomsforlife.com*.

We'll start your workout with a dynamic warm-up. Do each of these movements for about 45 seconds unless otherwise noted.

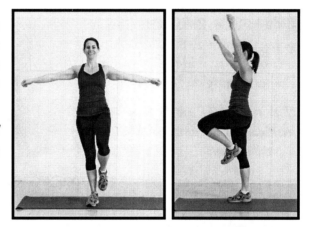

High Knee Steps with Arm Circles: Begin by making circular forward arm circles. Once you are doing that, incorporate a high knee march.

Tip: *Do some arm circles big and some small, and don't forget to make backward arm circles too.*

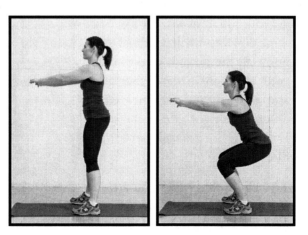

Bodyweight Squats: Feet should be about shoulder-width apart and toes pointed either straight ahead or at 11 and 1 o'clock. Put most of your weight in the mid- to back part of the foot and squat down as low as you can, trying to get your thighs parallel to the ground.

Tip: *If you are having a hard time getting low, put your hands out in front of your body to counterweight your butt. You can also try putting a book or magazine under your heels when you squat.*

Side-to-Side Lateral Shifting: Set your feet a bit wider than shoulder-width. Keep toes pointed straight ahead. Begin shifting side-to-side, feeling a stretch in the groin and inner thighs.

Tip: To increase the intensity, sit back more and put more weight in the heel, and sink the butt closer to the ground.

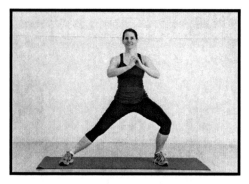

Side-to-Side Rotations: This is going to warm up the core (middle section). Twist side-to-side keeping the torso upright.

Tip: If you have a tight lower back, ease into this and start by just twisting a small amount.

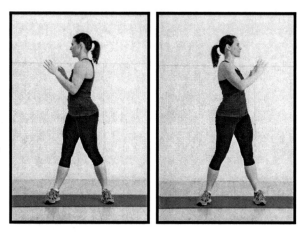

Total Body Circles: Begin with your hands above your head and, as you squat down, bring both arms down to the left side of your body. At the bottom of the squat, your arms are toward your feet, and as you stand the arms come around the right side of the body. Do five full circles and then switch direction.

Tip: To get an even better stretch, at the top of this movement, lift your heels off the ground and stand on your toes.

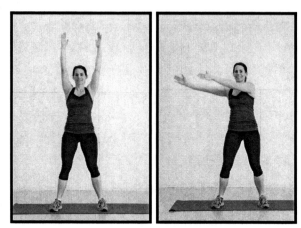

Stationary Skipping: Lift your left arm above your head and lift your right leg so that your knee is at waist height. In one smooth motion, reverse it, so that the right arm is lifted up and the left knee is at waist height.

Tip: If this is too hard, go back to a marching type motion, instead of a skip. To make it more intense, try to jump high with each skip.

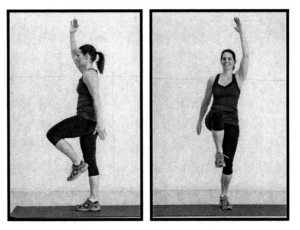

You should feel warm and be starting to break a sweat after this warm-up. Now let's move in to your full-body strength training workout. Do each exercise for one minute and move quickly to the next one. Once you've gone through all the exercises, take a short break (no more than a minute or two) and then go through the circuit one more time.

As you go through these exercises, remember to keep breathing. Exhale on the exertion part of the exercise—as you push the weight above your head, for example.

Seated Shoulder Press on Ball: Sit nice and tall on the stability ball and bring the dumbbells up to your shoulders, with palms facing forward. Press both arms up until the dumbbells nearly touch at the top, and then slowly lower back down to the shoulders.

Recommended weights for beginners: 10-pound dumbbells

Tip: If the shoulder press hurts your shoulders, don't lower the weight all the way back down to the shoulders. Stop a few inches above.

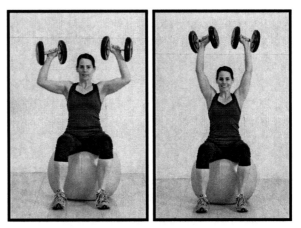

Push-Ups: Place your hands wider than your shoulders but in line with the shoulders/chest. Lower your chest toward the ground, stopping when your shoulder is at the same height as your elbow. Make sure to keep your abs pulled in, and maintain neutral alignment throughout the exercise.

Tip: If you can't do push-ups on your toes quite yet, try this instead: Start on your toes and lower your body as slowly as you can, until you collapse on the floor. Then drop your knees to the ground and push back up. Within no time, knees won't be necessary. To make push-ups more difficult, put your feet up on a chair or lift one leg.

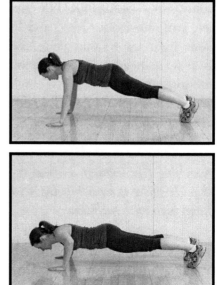

Ball Hip Raises: Lying with your back on the floor, place both feet on top of a stability ball. Press your heels into the ball and lift your butt up. Try to lift it up high enough that your knees, hips, and shoulders make a straight line. Lower back down until you almost touch the ground, then lift again.

Tip: If you are having trouble lifting the hips that high, try it without the ball. If this is too easy, lift one leg, and just use one leg to raise the hips.

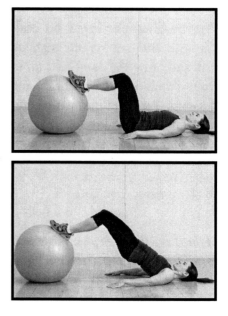

Dumbbell Bent Row on Ball: With feet wider than shoulder-width, stand behind the stability ball. Hold a dumbbell in one hand. Bend over and place the other hand on the ball, lengthening your spine and flattening out your back. Pull the dumbbell up toward your chest and give the upper back a squeeze, and then slowly lower back down. Keep back flat and try not to rotate the torso as you lift. Do 30 seconds with each arm.

Recommended weights for beginners: One 10- to 15-pound dumbbell

Tip: You can either have your elbow out or in; both are great and can add some variety.

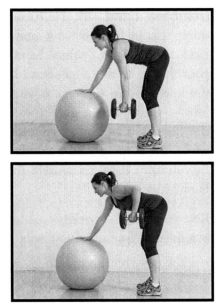

Rear Deltoid Raises: Feet shoulder-width apart, bend over, similar to the bent row, but without the ball in front of you. With a slight bend in your elbows, raise the dumbbells so that your arms are extended to the side. As you raise the weights, rotate your arms so that your thumbs are pointing up toward the ceiling. Slowly lower back down.

Recommended weights for beginners: 5-pound dumbbells

Tip: This is a great exercise to improve posture. It doesn't take much weight to feel it. Focus on getting a good squeeze between the shoulder blades at the top of the motion.

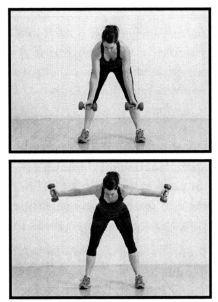

Dumbbell Dead Lift: Hold two dumbbells in front of your body, near your thighs, palms facing your thighs. With a slight bend in the knees, begin to bend at your hips, lowering the weights toward the floor. Go as low as you can while still keeping your back flat. As you come back up, squeeze the hamstrings and butt.

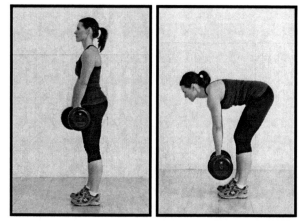

Recommended weights for beginners: 15-pound dumbbells

Tip: Dead lifts are one of the best exercises, but can be one of the most dangerous if the lower back isn't in the right position. Make sure that when you bend over, you aren't rounding the back; if you are, it will put too much stress on the lower back. Instead, stick your butt back, and lift your chest as you lower yourself. If you have tight hamstrings, you might only be able to lower down six inches. That is just fine.

> " The strength training is really hard physically, and it's a challenge, but it's like, 'OK, I can do anything for a minute. I can do this. I'll try my best for a minute.' It seems like such a doable thing."
> – Laura

Dumbbell Squats: Feet should be about shoulder-width apart. Holding the dumbbells by your sides, squat down in the same motion as described in the warm-up. Try to lower the butt to about knee height, keeping your knees behind your toes. Look straight ahead to maintain a neutral back.

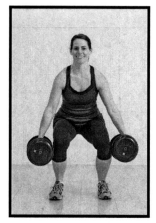

Recommended weights for beginners: 15- to 20-pound dumbbells

Tip: To make this more challenging, you can hold the dumbbells up by your shoulders instead of by your side. This will require more core strength.

Back Lunges: Hold dumbbells at your sides and take a moderate step backward. Then lower the body in a vertical motion, so that your back knee, which is bent, almost touches the ground. Also make sure the front knee is right above the heel, and not over the toe.

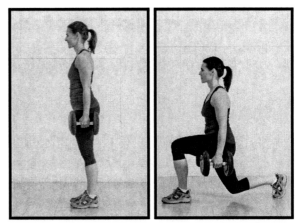

Recommended weights for beginners: 15- to 20-pound dumbbells

Tip: Lunges can cause problems for people with bad knees. If your knees get sore, don't go so deep into the lunge, or opt to do a step-up onto a bench instead of a lunge.

Once you've gone through this strength training circuit twice, it's time for burst cardio. You can choose the interval that works for you from the chart on page 112. I'd suggest you start with doing each of these exercises for one minute and resting for one to three minutes depending on how fatigued you are. Do each of these twice.

Squat Undercut Punches with Dumbbells: Feet should be a little wider than shoulder-width, arms bent and palms up. Hold a light dumbbell in each hand. Rotate your body to the right side while coming across the body with the left arm. Alternate sides.

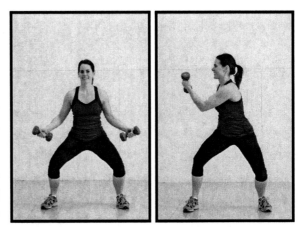

Tip: Focus on squeezing the oblique abs (side abs) as you twist and generate the power through the core and legs.

High Knee Punching: Similar to the skipping during the warm-up, but this time hold light dumbbells (5-pounders) in your hands. This exercise should be done very quickly and explosively. Make sure to get full range of motion on the shoulder presses.

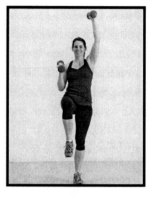

Tip: This exercise can feel awkward at first; don't get frustrated. With practice you will get it. If this is hard on the knees, go to a march instead of running in place.

Pretend Jump Rope: Feet about shoulder-width apart and hands by your side, start with small jumps while using your arms to pretend you are twirling a jump rope. Feel free to change it up and jump side-to-side or front and back.

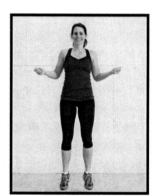

Tip: Make this fun by mixing it up. Try some jumps that are slower but bigger, while others are very short and quick.

With your heart pumping, it's time to focus on those core muscles.

Vacuum: Exhale all the air out of your lungs and then hold your breath. Forcefully draw your belly button in toward your spine in a sucking-in motion. Hold that for five to 10 seconds. Regain a normal breath and repeat five times.

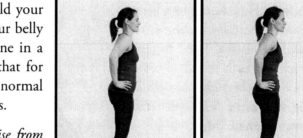

Tip: You can do this exercise from many different positions. Try lying on your back, on all fours, sitting in the car—however you would like. You should feel a drawing-in from very low, below the belly button, right above the pubic bone.

Front Plank: Forearms are on the ground and shoulders are positioned right above the elbows. Your abs are drawn in and your legs are contracted. Hold this position for 45 seconds while breathing naturally. Make sure the hips don't stick up too high or sag too low.

Tip: To make planks more challenging, lift a leg, or an arm, or the opposite leg and arm.

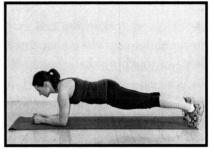

Side Plank: Lying on your side, stack your feet on top of each other and place your elbow under your shoulder. Lift the hips high, creating a long, straight profile. Hold for 30 seconds, then switch to the other side and hold that for 30 seconds.

Tip: If this is too hard, bend the bottom leg, place that knee on the floor, and lift the hips from there. If it is too easy, lift the top leg and hold.

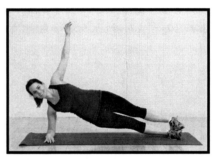

Swimmers: Lying on your belly, stretch the arms above the head and point the toes. Make the body as long as possible. Lift the opposite arm and leg and bring them back down, then move on to the other side. Do your best to get the fronts of your thighs off the floor as you kick with straight legs. Make sure to pull the belly in to support the back. Continue for 45 seconds.

Tip: To make this more interesting, bring the legs out wider, like you are trying to do the splits, and bring the arms out more to the sides, so you look more like a star.

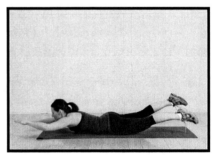

Back Extensions on the Ball: Lie across the ball facedown, with the ball at your pelvis and lower abdomen. Have your knees slightly bent, but not touching the ground. Hands should be by your ears with elbows out. Lower your upper body over the ball, reaching your head toward the floor. Then exhale, and engage your lower back muscles as you lift your head and chest. Only raise your head and chest until your body forms a straight line—don't overextend.

Tip: Many people have a hard time balancing on this one. Place your feet against a wall for extra stability if you are having a hard time.

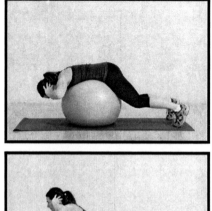

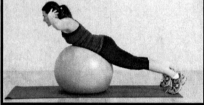

Ball Crunches: Lie across the stability ball with your lower back on the ball and reach your hands directly up toward the ceiling. Lift the hands up toward the ceiling by engaging the abs and crunching up. Draw the abs into the spine and exhale as you reach up. Slowly lower back down all the way, so that your shoulders touch the ball and the abdomen is fully stretched. Do 15 reps.

Tip: If this is hurting your lower back, put the ball up higher toward your mid- to upper back. If this is too easy, hold a dumbbell in your hands as you crunch up.

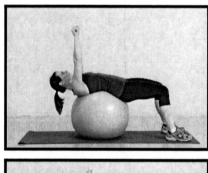

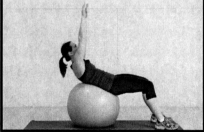

Oblique Ball Crunches: Same ball position as the regular crunches, but this time your hands are by your ears and your elbows are pointed out. Without moving the ball or your legs, crunch so that you bring your left shoulder toward your right hip. Lower back down to neutral and repeat on the other side. Do 20 reps (10 on each side).

Tip: To make this harder, you can hold a dumbbell underneath your chin.

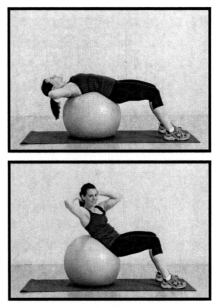

Congratulations, you are done with the "work" part of your workout! Do some stretching to reduce your risk of injury and muscle soreness. Hold each stretch for 20 to 30 seconds.

Downward Dog: While in a push-up position, stick your butt high in the air, and walk your hands toward your feet. Pull your chest in toward your thighs and open up your shoulders.

Tip: This is probably the best-known yoga move. It is supposed to be a resting pose, but I find it extremely challenging. To make it easier on your calves and hamstrings, bend a little at the knees and don't push your heels into the ground.

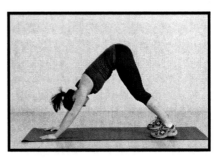

Upward Dog: From a push-up position, lift your chest and look up to the ceiling. Keep your shoulders pressed down. Sink the hips toward the ground while reaching the chest up. The tops of the feet should be on the ground.

Tip: If you are feeling pain in your lower back, don't lift the chest so high or drop the hips so low.

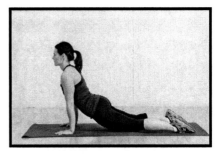

Overhead Triceps Stretch: Raise one arm over your head and bend at the elbow so that your hand is at the back of your neck. Place your other hand on the raised elbow and pull back a little bit.

Tip: Instead of using your other hand to pull, you can hold a light dumbbell to help pull the elbow back.

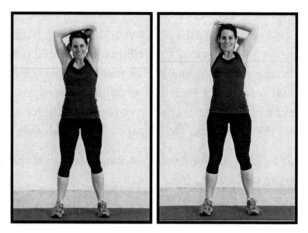

Chest Stretch: Interlock your hands behind your back and slowly raise your arms, feeling a stretch in your chest. Feel free to also hinge over at the waist for even more of a stretch.

Tip: Some people can't interlock their hands together behind their backs. If this is the case, hold on to a towel or have a friend pull your arms back.

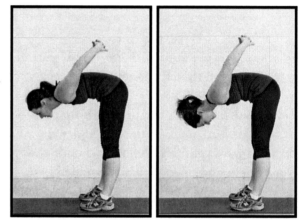

Hamstring Stretch: While standing, cross one leg over the other and reach your hands toward the floor. Go until you feel slight discomfort and then repeat on other leg.

Tip: To get an even more intense stretch, wrap your arms and hands behind your calves and knees, and try to bring the face toward the legs.

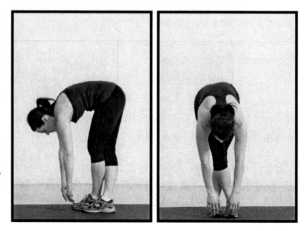

Full Body Reach: Stand on your tippy toes and reach as high as you can upward.

Tip: Pretend that there is a $100 bill right above your fingertips.

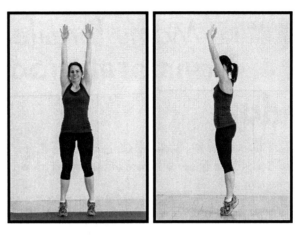

Glute Stretch: While lying on your back, cross one leg over the other at a 90-degree angle and pull your knee toward your body. Try to keep your lower back on the ground.

Tip: If you want an even greater stretch, have a friend stand in front of you and push your knee into your chest even more.

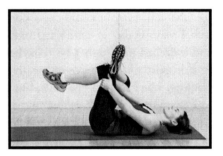

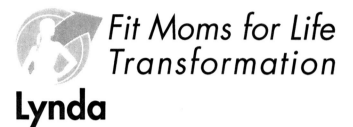

Fit Moms for Life Transformation

Lynda

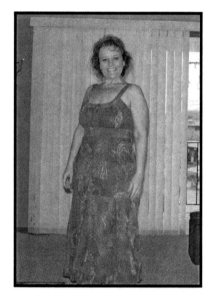

Lynda's transformation has been amazing, inside and out. Her efforts in Fit Fun Boot Camp have really paid off, and she is down to a size 14 from her high of a 24.

Lynda's story: "Last winter, my husband was deployed to Afghanistan. I took our son to Cancun for his 21st birthday and when we got the pictures back, I couldn't believe what I looked like. I knew I didn't want to look like that when my husband came home in December. I decided that March 1 was my day to start watching what I ate. I talked to my doctor and switched to a higher-protein diet, really cutting down on the carbs. I dropped about 10 pounds really fast just with that. Then I started walking. I lost 25 to 30 pounds, but by July, I noticed it wasn't coming off anymore. I wasn't pushing myself enough. I found Fit Fun Boot Camp online and thought it looked like fun. The first time I went, I thought they might have to leave me dead in the parking lot! But the instructors are so encouraging, and I just kept going.

Lynda, 42, mother of one. 5'4", 181 pounds. Lynda has lost 87 pounds so far doing my boot camps, after slowly putting on weight over the past 25 years. She's taken 37¾ inches from her body measurements and completely reversed her blood cholesterol levels.

"My husband came home from Afghanistan in December. I was at the airport to meet him, and he walked right past me. He didn't even recognize me. We had seen each other when he was on leave in May, but that was before I had started boot camp. I hadn't changed my hair or anything! I had to call out his name—he turned around and couldn't believe it was me.

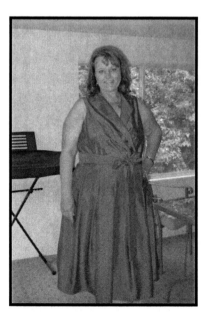

"My colleagues and friends can't believe the change in not only my personality and my looks, but also just the way I hold myself. I walk with more confidence. My head is up high."

Lynda's advice to you: "Take any first step. Start to walk. That's where I started—walking outside and not really pushing myself that hard. But just being able to walk three blocks without being out of breath was kind of big for me back then. You don't have to jump into an entire fitness routine from day one."

Read more of Lynda's story at *fitmomsforlife.com/lynda*.

Fit Moms for Life Transformation

Mary

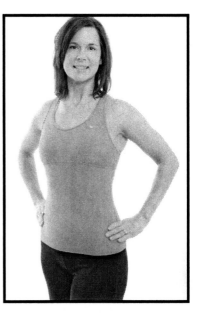

Mary has been coming to boot camp for over a year and has really changed the shape of her body. Even more exciting, she has started taking nutrition classes and is now coaching other women and sharing her passion for health and fitness.

Mary's story: "A little over a year ago, when I was approaching turning 40, I started Dustin's program. I just wanted to look better and feel better, and I knew that as I was aging, it was only going to get more difficult to lose weight and get into shape. I am now 41 years old and in the best shape of my life!

"When I started, I couldn't even do a push-up, and now I can easily do 20. My family is very active, and I can really tell how much stronger I am when I'm playing tennis, water-skiing, and downhill skiing. I even tried snowboarding and did my first sprint triathlon last fall.

"I wanted to share what I've learned with other people, so I started teaching weekly classes to help people learn how to live a healthier lifestyle through healthier eating and exercise. I'm coaching women who have been struggling with weight loss or poor eating habits. We focus on a specific topic every week. I've found that when people learn why we need to do all of these things and why things are good for your health or bad for your health, it has more of an impact. Coaching these other women is so rewarding, especially seeing the results they're getting from making healthier choices."

Mary, 41, mother of two. 5'6½", 139 pounds. Mary lost 15 pounds and went down two pants sizes once she started doing boot camps and learning about nutrition.

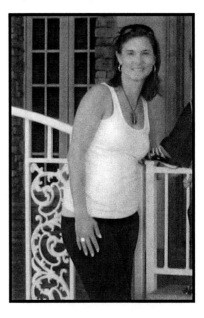

Mary's nutrition tips: "Eat more vegetables, organic if possible. That's the one thing most nutritionists agree on and what most people are lacking in their diet. Spend time on planning and preparing healthy food so that it's always on hand. I bring food with me wherever I go. I also have a mini refrigerator in my office at work. You just have to make the time to eat healthy."

Mary's advice to you: "Don't take your health for granted. You need to make your health your number one priority, which means spending the time and money it takes to improve it and maintain it."

Read more of Mary's story at *fitmomsforlife.com/mary*.

ENVIRONMENT: STAYING FIT FOR LIFE

"It's not only helping me and my health, but it's also carrying over to my family. My husband and my children are eating much better." – Mary

"Well, you know, you've got to change your diet, and you've got to exercise more. But I think it's really important to have either a community or a higher power that you're getting strength from, because you do have to dig deep. It could be God, or boot camp, or the universe.... But if you don't have some source for that strength, you're going to be back up at those 240 pounds before you even realize what happened." – Nancy

I've gone through the nuts and bolts of what you need to eat and how you need to exercise in my program. But as I said in the beginning, it's not just about eating right and exercising. The other pillars of fitness are mindset, which we addressed in the first section of the book, and environment, which we're getting to now. From the people you spend time with to what you do in your free time with your family, the environment you live in can determine whether you will truly be able to transform your body and your life, and maintain those positive changes over time.

In 2010, I interviewed two contestants from season seven of *The Biggest Loser*, Kristin and Cathy. (You can watch the interview at *fitmomsforlife.com/biggestloser*.) They had gone into the show weighing close to 300 pounds each, and they had each lost more than 100 pounds on the show. They told me how they had to create a new environment for themselves when they got home from *The Biggest Loser*, because when they were obese, they had created one that supported their behaviors. They knew what brands of cars would accommodate their bellies and chests. They knew what restaurants to go to not just because they liked the food, but also because they knew there were tables in those restaurants where they could fit. They knew which stores to go to where they could park close to the doors. They had actually spent a lot of energy creating an environment that made it comfortable for them to keep ignoring their health, whether they did it consciously or not. When they got home again, they realized they had to put just as much energy into re-creating their environment in a way that would support their new healthy lifestyles. They have new routines around going to the gym every day. They choose restaurants now based on where they know they can get a healthy meal – and they don't have to worry any more about whether they'll fit at the table. These are the changes that will help them maintain their weight loss, because otherwise they would slip right back into their old unhealthy habits.

Of course, your environment isn't just about you improving your own health and fitness. It's about raising a healthy family and being part of a healthy community. You have the power to make your home a healthy environment and teach your children to make positive choices for their health and fitness. Chapter 10 includes a lot of great tips on how to do that. You also have the power to help other women (and men) make the same changes in their lives. Just as much as I want you to create an environment that supports your healthy behaviors, I also want you to make the same kind of transformation possible for other people. Find people who will be part of your supportive community, and you can be part of theirs, too. In Chapter 11, I will go into more detail about my vision for Fit Moms for Life communities of women who are working on putting themselves first, eating well, feeding their families well, and exercising with a combination of strength training and burst training to get into their best shape ever. Finally, in Chapter 12, we'll visualize what your transformation is going to look like, and you'll be ready to go.

Fit Mom, Fit Family

Every parent wants to raise healthy children, but many parents seem to struggle to do it these days. I believe it all comes down to setting a good example for your kids. If kids don't see their parents making healthy choices, how are they going to learn to do it themselves? How can you expect them to want to be active if they see you on the couch watching two hours of TV every night? Why wouldn't they crave fast food if you're taking them to McDonald's every time you're out and about? How are your kids supposed to choose to eat fruits and vegetables if you don't have them readily available, you don't serve them with meals, and you don't eat them in front of your kids? If you give them the information, expose them to healthy eating and exercise, and show them how you incorporate those things into your life, they'll have the tools they need to make good choices for themselves. My mom did an excellent job of this. She was 33 years old when she had me, and she had three more kids pretty quickly after that. She was able to take off her pregnancy weight with each child. She was always talking to us about what we ate, asking, "Why is this healthy for us, and why is this other thing not healthy?" It definitely made a big impression on me and is part of what led me to do what I do now.

In this chapter, I'll give you some tips for teaching your kids to be healthy eaters, whether you have young kids right now or older kids who have started to learn some bad habits. I'll also go over how to keep your kids active and physically fit. I'm not a parent and I'm not an expert on children—but I have seen what worked in my family growing up and what works for hundreds of my clients who are moms.

I do have one precaution before we get into this, though: We never want to teach kids to associate healthy eating and exercise with losing weight or dieting. We want them to learn how to keep themselves healthy; the last thing we need is to get our young kids obsessed with weight loss and how their bodies look. There is enough of that out there already. I don't like when moms talk about needing to lose weight in front of their kids—and I really don't like when I hear a mom tell her kid, "Eat this so you don't get fat," or especially, "Eat this because you're getting fat." Talk about it in terms of health and energy and how they will feel, and what their bodies will be able to do if they eat well and exercise.

Developing Healthy Eating Habits in Your Kids

I'll go through specific tips for kids of different ages below, but a few things are true for any age. Most nutritionists and child development experts follow a philosophy regarding children's eating that's called the "division of responsibility."[1] The idea is that the parent's job is to provide healthy options at the appropriate times, and the child's job is to decide how much of it to eat—or whether to eat it at all. I talk to a lot of moms who cater to exactly what the kid wants and get really frustrated if their child doesn't eat enough. At the other extreme, a lot of parents resort to bribes or punishments to try to get kids to eat what they're served. None of that helps kids learn to listen to their own hunger and satiety cues, and it doesn't help them learn healthy eating habits. (If you're having dessert, which I hope is not every day, don't make your kids "earn" it by eating past the point of fullness.)

The moms I work with have told me this is easier said than done at times! But the idea is that you set the schedule and offer healthy choices at regular meal and snack times. The kids eat from what is served, in whatever quantity they need. If they don't eat much at one meal, they'll catch up and eat more next time. Most kids will get the right amount of calories and the right breakdown of nutrients this way. You will also avoid eating becoming a power struggle, which can be bad news for your relationship with your child and for your child's future eating habits.

It's so important to educate your kids about healthy food. Even at a really young age, you can start talking about things like where food comes from and how different foods make our bodies feel. As kids get older, you can start to get more into things like why it's important to have protein with every meal and what are healthy sources of the different nutrients we need. You want to equip your child to make good choices when they are in charge of their own eating, but that likely won't happen if they don't understand the reasons behind what is "healthy" and what is not.

Another strategy that you can use throughout your kids' lives is to involve them in selecting and preparing the food, in a way that is age-appropriate. Very young kids might just choose which kind of fruit they're having with their snack. You can also give them tasks in the grocery store, like holding the list or looking for certain foods as you go through the store. (If you have multiple children, try to occasionally go grocery shopping with just one child, so you can make the most of it as a

---

1 Satter, Ellyn. Child of Mine: <u>Feeding with Love and Good Sense</u>. Boulder, CO: Bull Publishing, 2000.

learning experience.) As they get older, they can take on more responsibility in the kitchen, like planning meals, making the grocery list, helping with the shopping, and eventually cooking for the family. My mom sometimes made me responsible for making a dinner for the family. I would have to go through her cookbooks and find a recipe that looked good. We would write down the ingredients we didn't have and go to the grocery store to get them. Next I would help prepare and cook the meal, and then finally serve it to the whole family. Not only did this teach me how to cook and what ingredients were in different recipes, but it gave me a sense of ownership for the meal that I made, and it made me appreciate what went into creating a healthy dinner for the family every night.

> " The boys are older now, but when they were younger, they would see the effort I put into making a great, nutritionally balanced meal. Now that they're older and living on their own, they try to do that too."
> – Patrice

Getting started: Advice for mothers of infants and toddlers. Right when your child is born is the best time to start raising a healthy eater.[2] The best things you can do from the beginning are to breastfeed, if you can, and to feed the baby on demand. Breastfed babies stop eating when they're full, more so than bottlefed—maybe because nursing is hard work (for the baby) compared to drinking from a bottle, or maybe because parents will keep giving a bottle until it's empty. Breastfeeding may also help a baby get used to different tastes, because the milk will change slightly depending on what the mother eats. Feeding on demand, rather than on a schedule, also helps the baby recognize what hunger feels like and learn to eat when hungry.

Of course, you can also raise a healthy eater if you use formula, or if your baby drinks expressed milk from a bottle, or is fed on a set schedule. Watch carefully for signs that your baby has had enough to eat (for example, slowing down his sucking or finding something more interesting to look at). Try taking the bottle out of his mouth at that point and asking whether he's full. If he's distressed about the bottle being taken away, continue feeding; but if he isn't, he is probably full, and you should stop feeding regardless of how much is left in the bottle.

Whether you breastfeed or use formula, hold off on introducing solid foods until your baby is six months old. (Recent research indicates that introducing solid food earlier than four months is linked with obesity later in childhood for formula-fed babies in particular.[3]) Once you do introduce solid food, don't spend too long on pureed food. You can make a gradual transition to lumpier foods, and then mashed-up and cut-up table food, so that your baby is eating what you eat by his or her first birthday. It's even easier to make that gradual transition if you make your own baby food, which I really recommend. Most of the commercial baby food available is highly processed and bland. It's no wonder some kids object to "real" food when they taste it for the first time! Making your own baby

2 Dwyer, Johanna T., et al. "Feeding Infants and Toddlers Study 2008: Progress, Continuing Concerns, and Implications." Journal of the American Dietetic Association 110.12 (2010): S60-S67.
3 Huh, SY, et al. "Timing of Solid Food Introduction and Risk of Obesity in Preschool-Aged Children." Pediatrics 127.3 (2011): e544-51.

food is as easy as cooking, pureeing or mashing, and adding the right amount of liquid. You can even make it in large batches and freeze it in ice cube trays so you have a freezer full of serving-size food cubes when you need them. Making your own is also much better for your grocery bill.

Once your baby is eating solid foods, introduce a variety of vegetables, fruits, and grains. They may or may not eat everything you offer—but remember that some kids may need to be exposed to something as many as 10 times before they will eat it. So be patient and don't get too bent out of shape about it. Remember, your job is to provide the healthy options. As long as your child is eating a variety of foods, don't get hung up on whether she eats any one particular food.

As you get into the toddler years, many kids get pickier and eat less in general. For one thing, they're not growing as fast as they did in the first year of life, so they actually don't need as many calories. There is also a theory that toddlers' caution about putting anything new or unknown in their mouths may protect them from eating something poisonous when they're first walking and encountering things without their parents. From an evolutionary perspective, it makes sense that toddlers are picky. And some studies have shown that even when parents think their toddlers aren't eating anything, they are getting the nutrients and calories they need.

It may help to know that kids' later eating habits tend to reflect the foods they were exposed to when they were young, not just what they actually ate. So resist the temptation to become a short-order cook. Don't start cooking separate meals for your picky toddler. Serve family meals that include at least one thing you know each child will eat, and let them find what they need from that. (One author suggests serving good bread with every meal—and being okay with it if a child chooses to eat just the bread.)

Making changes or keeping up the good work: Advice for mothers of older kids. With older kids who may already have some bad eating habits in place, it can be a little harder to implement healthy eating, but it's definitely still possible.

The most important thing you can do for a child of any age is to be a good example! They will see that you're eating healthy, eating often, and having the right portion sizes, drinking lots of water, and doing all of those things I talked about in the nutrition section. You know they'll certainly notice if you aren't doing those things while you're telling them they should!

At the same time, we talked about cheat meals in the nutrition section, and I think that's something you should teach your kids, too. They should know that you're not striving for perfection with your eating, but just making healthier choices, and giving yourself the occasional cheat meal or cheat day. Then they can learn to do the same, so they allow themselves to enjoy special occasions and treats without feeling guilty, and just focus on making the healthy choices most of the time.

If you have made some poor choices in the way you have fed your kids and yourself up until now, and you're planning to make some drastic changes, don't try to change everything at once, at least not for your kids. Make the changes gradually. Start with incorporating a vegetable into your dinner—or actually sitting down as a family to eat dinner if you haven't been doing that. If you were having dessert every single night, start to switch

> " My kids watch every single bite I take. When I would sneak a cookie, they were both right there, and they both wanted a cookie, too. You're a role model for your children."
>
> – Nancy

that out with fruit a couple days a week. Don't change everything all at once on your kids—this isn't a choice they're making, so it's only fair to give them some time to get used to it.

Again, if you're making these changes with older kids, you have to talk to them about what you're doing and why. They're definitely going to notice, and they may not like the changes. If you've been making them a grilled cheese sandwich for dinner every night for six years, they're not going to respond well to suddenly having to eat what everyone else is eating. So explain what you're doing. Be reasonable about it, but make it clear that the whole family is making changes to be healthier, and they will have to get used to it.

There are a couple books out about how to sneak vegetables into food for kids. Now, from a nutritional standpoint, that's great because you get the vitamins and nutrients from the veggies. However, from a practical standpoint, you're not teaching your kids to eat those healthy foods. So if you are really struggling to get your kids to eat enough vegetables, sneaking them in is certainly better than nothing, but you don't want to do that forever or at the expense of helping your kids develop healthy eating habits based upon actual whole foods that they can see.

Another way to get kids to start eating better is to make it fun. Let your kids have fun with healthy food. You can cut things up into special shapes, give kids vegetable sticks to dip into hummus or a ranch-style dip made with Greek yogurt, or set up a salad bar or taco bar for them to put together their own meal. Put small bites on toothpicks. If it makes your kids want to eat it, why not? The other idea that goes with this is to make eating healthy convenient. Stock your cupboards with healthy snack options and have fresh fruit and vegetables around for your kids to eat.

> " At first, my kids were saying, 'What? This doesn't taste like it's supposed to.' But I explained to them why we're eating this way and what this is and now it's what they know."
>
> – Jody

Starting a little garden in the backyard can be a good way to teach kids where our food comes from and that healthy options can be delicious. It is hard to top a fresh sugar snap pea or a ripe garden tomato! When they've put in the effort to grow the vegetables, they become more interested in eating them.

As your kids get older, there are a couple of things you can do to help them continue to make healthy choices at school. The first thing is to pack their lunches. Make it a family activity in the evening for everyone to pack what they're taking to school and work the next day, choosing from healthy options. If they're going to eat school lunch, talk to them about what the healthier options are and how to choose a meal that's going to help them stay alert and energetic for the rest of the day. Finally, if you're passionate about healthy food in schools, get involved in advocacy to make school lunches better for all kids.

Keeping Your Kids Active

Just like with getting your kids to eat healthy, keeping your kids active and fit is mostly a question of role modeling. As with all habits, the sooner you start, the easier it will be to make your kids lifelong exercisers and active people. That said, it's never too late to make a change.

Especially for younger kids, your goal is not to get them to "exercise" but just to be active throughout their day. Climbing a ladder and sliding down a slide, jumping up and down to music, going for a walk around the neighborhood, or trudging up a hill to go sledding provide all the exercise most toddlers and preschoolers need. As your kids get older, they might start to show more interest in sports, gymnastics, and other organized forms of exercise. That's great, but you still want to keep a focus on staying active. Be the kind of family that goes for a bike ride instead of watching a movie on a warm summer evening. Make sure your kids spend some time playing outside every day. Limit their television, computer, and video game time and get them moving instead. Jody told me that in her house, they even incorporate physical activity when they're watching TV. She, her husband, and her kids will do planks during commercials. They try to hold a front plank for one or two commercials, and then hold a side plank for one commercial on each side.

> " You have to shift gears into thinking about being active all the time. Like with my kids, if we want to spend a little time together, I'll say 'Hey, let's go take the dogs for a walk.' Or we'll go hiking, or go for a bike ride."
>
> – Jane

Another great idea is to involve your kids in your exercise. My *BabyTone* DVD shows moms ways to exercise with their babies—it solves the childcare problem that so many moms have when their kids are little and lets your child learn right away that exercise is part of life. If your kids are older, don't always wait until they're asleep to exercise. Let them join you. You can have wall-sit contests and do other exercises that are age-appropriate for them. I don't encourage you to do this all the time, because you won't get as good of a workout yourself when you're focusing on your kids, but it is very important that they see you doing it and having fun. Kids just want to move around and play, so the more fun you can make it, the better.

As for kids working out, there are a lot of misconceptions out there. The bottom line is that it's perfectly safe for them to exercise and even do strength training with light weights. I've gone to a few seminars with Avery Faigenbaum, who specializes in adolescent training. (See his and Wayne Westcott's book, *Youth Strength Training*, for more information.) They've found that strength training is not dangerous for kids of any age. It's not going to stunt their growth or anything like that. There are a couple things to be aware of, though. Of course, kids need lighter weights. You don't need them maxing out or straining to lift anything. Body-weight exercises like push-ups and planks are great for kids to work on coordination and balance. Learning to use slow and controlled motion and proper form is critical. With teenagers, there are some additional considerations. Teenage girls really benefit from strength training because it will help them build bone density, as I mentioned earlier. So, encouraging that is a great idea with your daughters. You've got to watch teenage boys if they're working out without any adults and trying to out-lift each other. That's when accidents can happen, especially with bench pressing. If you've got a weight bench in your house, keep a close eye on what your older kids are doing with it. With appropriate supervision, strength training and exercise in general are safe and healthy for kids, and I encourage you to help your kids develop that habit early.

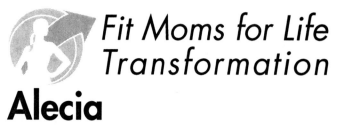

Fit Moms for Life Transformation

Alecia

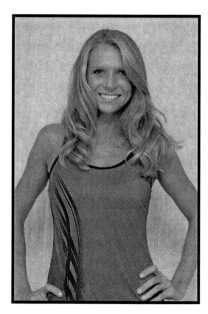

Alecia is probably the fittest mom I have worked with. She is a great example of someone who was already pretty fit but was still able to transform her body and get into even better shape through lifting heavy weights and burst training.

Alecia's story: "I was four months into my second pregnancy when I started Dustin's program. I was in pretty good shape and had been doing a lot of cardio before, but I could feel the difference right away when I started lifting heavy weights in Dustin's program. I think before I was skinny fat; now I'm skinny fit.

"While I was pregnant, I really had to watch and listen to my body and pay close attention to how I was feeling. Some days I could do a lot, and some days I had to take it easy and modify some things. I worked out up until the week before I had my daughter. I felt a lot better in that pregnancy than I did in my first one—I looked better and was less puffy. I was borderline hypoglycemic with my first pregnancy, and getting educated about nutrition really helped me keep that under control the second time around.

"After participating in Dustin's programs for two years, I actually gained about three pounds, but I lost a lot of body fat and went down two sizes. I thought I was strong before, but now I'm much stronger and a whole lot faster. I've toned up my stomach, arms, and back."

Alecia's current goals: "I'd like to run another marathon and train for an Ironman, but that's a few years off. I became certified as a personal trainer this year, and I'm also training to be a birth doula."

Alecia's exercise tips: "Find a friend to work out with who will keep you accountable. I want to get faster and just try new things, so my good friend and I find crazy fitness challenges to do together. And don't be nervous that other people are judging you when you go to work out. Everybody is concerned about themselves. They're not paying attention to how other people look. Just seek other people out so you have support."

Read more of Alecia's story at *fitmomsforlife.com/alecia,* and work out with her on the *BabyTone* DVD.

Alecia, 29, mother of two. 5'9", 140 pounds. Alecia went from a size 8 to a size 4 and reduced her body-fat percentage from 18 percent to 12 percent within a year after starting my program, when she was four months pregnant with her second child.

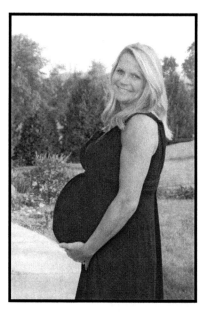

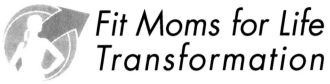

Fit Moms for Life Transformation

Patrice

Patrice is a woman who has not let her physical limitations stop her from changing her life. She's used my DVDs to lose weight and improve her strength and balance.

Patrice's story: "I have back problems that have gotten in the way of my efforts to get in shape in the past. I have rods and spinal fusion from back surgery that make me very stiff. I have some arthritis and bursitis, as well. I also have spinal stenosis, which makes my feet and legs numb. That throws off my balance and makes a lot of exercise challenging. I started using Dustin's *Fit Moms for Life* and *Got Core* DVDs about a year ago. It's been a challenge to find the happy medium between pushing myself enough but not pushing myself so hard that I would injure something. But I think I've got that now, because I'm getting stronger.

"I have gained strength and lost weight, and my back is doing better. I have less pain and stiffness. I feel like my posture has improved, and I don't lose my balance as much. This winter I was more able to catch myself when I started to slip on the ice, whereas in the past I would have just fallen down. I have a lot more energy, too. I feel more confident about myself. I'm able to do more things. I just feel that I'm handling myself better. I'm happier and probably calmer. And people are noticing."

Patrice's exercise tips: "If you have a health issue or a physical challenge, instead of getting wrapped up in what you can't do, focus more on what you can do. For example, I can't do a lot of the cardio because it's too high-impact. But I always watch that part of the DVD to see if I can do some of it, and if so, great. If not, can I alter it? And then as you get stronger, you can go back and see if you're able to do things that you couldn't do before. I couldn't do the push-ups when I started, but now I can. You get such a good feeling when you realize the gains you've made."

Read more of Patrice's story at *fitmomsforlife.com/patrice*.

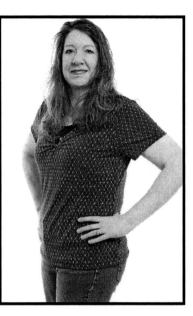

Patrice, 43, two grown stepchildren.
5'8", 172 pounds.
Patrice has lost 23 pounds and made fantastic gains in addressing some physical challenges she faces.

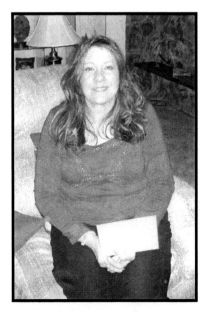

Creating Your Fitness Community

Women are great at getting together around shared interests on a regular basis. A lot of moms are in playgroups, book clubs, or church groups. They attend house parties to support other moms' businesses, they organize "Moms' Night Out" for everyone in the preschool class, or they get together with the other moms in their neighborhood to play Bunco. It sounds like fun, but I still see a lack of deep, authentic relationships, especially when it comes to sharing fitness and health. My vision is for moms to create groups that center around healthy lifestyles, supporting each other to make the right choices for themselves and their families.

Community: The Missing Piece of the Fitness Puzzle

If you're making the changes I suggest but your environment isn't supportive of them, it's going to be an uphill battle. It's hard to keep motivated for the long term if you're fighting against what everyone around you considers to be "normal" or if you don't have anyone to share the ups and downs of your fitness journey. That's why I'm so pumped about the community aspect of *Fit Moms for Life*. I can give you a workout plan and an eating plan, and you can be excited about it and follow it for a while, but for it to really stick, you need to find people who will support you and keep you accountable.

> *I know it is really annoying to be around people who are exercising because that's all they want to talk about. I'm one of them now."*
>
> – Aimee

Community is a very powerful influence on human behavior, and that influence can be positive or negative. We all have the innate desire to be part of a group and not to be left out of what others are doing. For example, I'm a trainer and I tend to hang out with other trainers—a lot of healthy people. My co-workers are all trainers, and my girlfriend is a trainer. If I were to start slacking off, not exercising, eating poorly, and gaining weight, I would be going against the norms of my group. Whether any of them said anything or not, it wouldn't take long before I would catch myself and get back on track.

Unfortunately, if you don't have that kind of healthy peer group, then trying to get healthy can actually be what makes you feel like an outsider. You start turning down invitations to go out to unhealthy meals, or you're skipping happy hour to go work out, or you'd rather talk about the amazing workout you did this morning than whatever was on TV last night. You're going against the norms of your group—and you might not find a lot of support. In the worst-case scenario, you're going to find that unhappy, unhealthy, overweight people are not going to let you escape to the happy, healthy, and fit category. I've seen it many, many times. They'll try to sabotage you, whether they know they're doing it or not, and I'm sorry to say it, but for the most part they will succeed if they have the numbers on their side.

> " *You definitely need a support system. People who are working out with you every morning, who will miss you when you're gone—that was big for me early on—or just people who are going to ask you how it's going and hold you accountable."*
>
> – Patty H.

Recently at one of my boot camp parties, I talked with a mom who is one of my fittest clients. Her whole life oozes with healthiness. For Christmas she visited her in-laws, who are on the opposite end of the health spectrum. She described Christmas dinner as all "fair food"—meaning food you would find at a fair, some of the worst around. She brought some of her own food and went for a three-mile run outside every day while she was there. She told me about the dirty looks she got and the mean jabs the extended family made toward her. It's a good thing she has a very strong, healthy support group that she sees most days and that the negative influences only come around the holidays.

Making big changes in ourselves sometimes requires changing the communities in which we participate. I'm not saying you need to cut off all your friendships and start from scratch—but you have to find some way to build support for what you're doing and cut down on the influence of people who don't want you to change or aren't going to support what you're doing. It could start with just having one workout partner—either someone else from within your existing social group who also wants to change or someone new. That's the minimum you need. The more support you can get, the better, but you need at least one person who's going to believe in you, be on the same page, and hold you to a different standard.

My Vision: Fit Moms for Life Communities

My vision is to have one million moms in the *Fit Moms for Life* community by the end of 2015. There will be a lot of different ways moms can be part of it, but my goal is that at least half a million of these moms will be plugged in to local workout-oriented support groups. There won't necessarily be certified trainers involved, although that may occur in the future. The community will grow mainly through individual moms embracing the *Fit Moms for Life* philosophy and approach, and putting together their own groups.

For instance, a mom hears about *Fit Moms for Life* and decides to start a group. She gathers her friends, or posts something on a social networking site to recruit other moms, or gets her kids' school or her church to sponsor a group. They might meet at her house, at a school or a church, or outside in a park. They get together on a regular basis—once, twice, or three times a week for some groups, maybe as little as every couple of weeks for other groups. When they get together, they exercise together, probably doing strength training and burst training following my program. They also have some discussion to get to know each other and build up all the components of a good support group, which I'm going to describe below. Between meetings they keep each other accountable for eating well and exercising using the *Fit Moms for Life* DVDs or another program. When people start to backslide or become inconsistent, the group is there to remind them why they're there and to encourage them to come back.

> " You never know who is out there just looking for a little inspiration, a little support, someone to point them in the right direction. And because they are looking to you for advice, for help—it helps you in return!"
> – Patty M.

The idea is to get to know each other at a deeper level, sharing the successes as well as the challenges they experience, and helping each other overcome the challenges. I envision *Fit Moms for Life* groups developing authentic relationships that go way beyond fitness—these become the friends you can count on to be there for you in good times and bad.

In addition to the local groups, an online component with a membership area allows women to talk to other moms doing the same thing in other parts of the country and the world. Even though I see the local support groups as the most important part of it, the online component helps to build closeness between the local groups and keep the movement growing. Just like any good support group, the international *Fit Moms for Life* community will need to grow to stay vibrant, and that will happen as women get results. As individuals and groups attain positive results and are motivated to share those success stories with people still struggling, the *Fit Moms for Life* worldwide community will grow exponentially.

As this book goes to press, I am planning the first international *Fit Moms for Life* convention, which will become a regular event. *Fit Moms for Life* conventions are opportunities for everyone to come together, meet each other in person, exercise together, learn advanced nutrition strategies, and become more motivated by top speakers from all over the world. *Fit Moms for Life* is becoming a powerful community, supporting authentic relationships with a focus on fitness. By now I hope you have decided that YOU want to become a *Fit Mom for Life* and a part of this growing movement. I can't do it without you!"

What's Happening With Fit Moms for Life Communities

Fit Moms for Life communities are springing up all over the country. Thousands of women subscribe to the monthly DVD program, with many of them starting their own *Fit Moms for Life* groups in their communities. (I got to meet members of some *FMFL* communities in North Dakota—read more about what Patty M. and Kim are doing with their groups on page 158.) I have developed a curriculum for groups to follow, with the basic structure for the meetings, nutritional lessons, and exercise lessons, so that a mom who wants to run her own group can pick it up and get going, equipped with the basic knowledge she needs and the resources for more information. You can also access materials on how to market your group, how to find a free location to use, and how to get other moms involved. Check *fitmomsforlife.com* to see what's happening with *Fit Moms for Life* communities now and get involved.

Components of an Effective Support Group

There are many components to an effective support group, whatever its purpose. Here are the important aspects of a *Fit Moms for Life* community:

Accountability. We all need other people to hold us accountable for our actions. For whatever reason, we're good at letting ourselves down and we're good at making excuses for failing to do what we intended or what we said we were going to do. It's much harder to not follow through when we've told someone else what our goals are, and said what steps we're going to take. Your fitness community can help with accountability regarding how you eat, how often you exercise, and what you accomplish.

Positivity. One of the biggest reasons I love my job as a trainer is that I'm able to interact with people who are really trying to be their best and be positive. I get to be surrounded by positive energy all day, which is awesome. You need to find a group of people who will be positive. Yes, there are going to be challenges. You'll have weight-

> " I like to work out with friends when I can. But in lieu of that, just to have accountability, I sometimes tell my husband or a friend, 'I'm going to work out today.'"
> – Becky

loss plateaus, and personal issues will slow you down at times. Surrounded by a positive group of people, you can get through those times and even spin some of your challenges into positives. I think you will find that the Law of Attraction is at work here: If you're thinking positively, you will attract positive energy.

Openness. We're so technologically advanced today, with more ways to communicate than ever before. Unfortunately, despite all the status updates, tweets, and chats, I think many people lack deep, authentic relationships. Do you have someone you can talk to

> *If one of us isn't in the mood, we feed off each other's motivation and get back on track."*
> – Kim

about your deepest, darkest secrets, or your biggest challenges, or most embarrassing experiences or feelings, knowing they're going to respect you and be open to what you have to say? A lot of people don't have that. Openness within the group is paramount, allowing people to talk about their struggles and their triumphs. Hand in hand with that, everyone needs to have a sense that what they say in that kind of relationship is confidential and no one is going to blab about it.

Authenticity. Being real, letting down our walls, and just being authentic with other people goes along with my last point. Getting beyond casual chitchat and actually finding out how someone is doing, or why they're doing great or not so great today, you can develop much more meaningful relationships. In a group built around authentic relationships, one person can share her current struggles and the rest of the group can help her work through it.

Structure. Groups need structure to keep them on-task and to ensure everyone's time is respected. Whether it's a framework for a group exercise session or an agenda for a meeting, a *Fit Moms for Life* community needs to have a specific plan of action and stick to it to be effective.

Passion. Each person in the group should be there with a clear purpose, and everyone should be passionate about what they're doing. Everyone in your *Fit Moms for Life* community should be someone who wants to be healthier, happier, fitter, and more positive. They probably want to live longer and have more energy. Be clear about your group's purpose and make sure everyone is trying to live out that purpose.

> *It is awesome to be around other women for 45 minutes a day without your kids, getting to know them and exchanging tips. It really makes you feel less alone."*
> – Aimee

Camaraderie. Camaraderie is what allows you to keep going during a tough workout, or what convinces you to get back on the eating plan after you broke all the rules on vacation. Whether it's through positive encouragement or friendly competition, the group energy is what's going to keep you going. If no one's watching, it's too easy to quit when things get a little bit challenging. My clients who come to boot camps and other group classes always talk about how important the camaraderie is to them, and I want everyone in a *Fit Moms for Life* community to experience it, too.

Viral aspect. For any group to prosper over time, it needs to be dynamic. If all these other things are put in place, you're going to be getting results and excited to tell others about them. Hopefully, that will bring more people into the group. You want to have a routine, but you also need new energy and new people coming in to keep things exciting and interesting. I really feel that if a group isn't growing in numbers or closeness, it's dying. You need to be achieving the kind of results that attract new members to keep your community strong.

> " Women just like me are out there, looking for exactly what I was looking for. It's nice to get together with other moms and women who share the same frustrations, like time constraints and muffin tops. It's also very rewarding to watch someone get excited about results and see the positive changes that exercise can make."
>
> – Kim

Fun. Your *Fit Moms for Life* group should also be fun, or what's the point? It should be fun to get together and share successes and struggles and work through them. It should be fun to work out alongside each other and push each other to do your best. Getting to know people at a deep level and learning that you can count on them should be fun and gratifying, too. Without fun, you're not going to keep people involved and you're certainly not going to grow. As my client Nancy put it, "This is the hardest fun I've ever had."

Benefits of a Fitness Community

Once you start developing your *Fit Moms for Life* community, you're going to realize great benefits from it. Whether you're in a group of two or a group of 25, these are some of the things you can expect to get out of it:

Accountability for eating well. I've already talked about food journals a couple times. Keeping a food journal is really valuable in and of itself. However, if you then share your food journal with another person and let them give you some feedback, it takes it to another level entirely. Knowing that someone else is going to look at your food journal is going to make you think twice about eating something you know you shouldn't. Your partner might also look at your journal and notice something you're not seeing yourself.

Sharing resources. There are a lot of resources your group can share with each other to make exercise and healthy eating fit into your day. For example, figuring out what to do with your kids while you exercise is always a challenge, but if you work out with a group, you can find ways to share childcare responsibilities. Maybe one person watches the kids while the others work out, and you rotate who is on childcare duty. You can also share transportation to get to your workout or a group meeting. Carpooling is a great way to get a little extra time together and save on gas. It also adds some accountability, because if someone's waiting for you to pick her up, you're not going hit the snooze button and skip the workout! Equipment is another thing you can share. Maybe you don't have all the equipment you want or need for the workouts, but everyone can bring what they have. You can also share things like recipes, inspirational videos you've found online, or whatever it may be. Sharing all these types of resources helps bring your group closer together and benefits everyone in it.

Partner exercises. I absolutely love partner exercises. For one of my programs, shown on the *Ultimate Buddy Boot Camp* DVDs, we use each other's body weight for resistance. There are a lot of cool things you can do with a partner that you can't do on your own. I think when you sweat together, there's a certain bond that's formed that's different from other friendships. You're in the moment together, and you're encouraging each other, and you're pushing each other to reach new levels of strength and fitness. So you're building the camaraderie through exercise, too.

> *Without the carpooling, there would be no way. The carpool factor is huge for me. When you know you've got people out there waiting to be picked up, you can't make excuses."*
> – Trish

Celebrating successes. When you're working out with a group and sharing all these experiences, you can truly celebrate each other's accomplishments. Especially if you don't have a lot of fit people in your life, it might feel like you're just bragging when you tell them you've lost 10 pounds or you just dropped two minutes on your mile time. Some people don't want to hear about that, and they might even say negative things and bring you down. You need to have people who will celebrate those successes with you. I think this is true not only for your fitness successes, but also in other areas of your life. I'm in a group for personal trainers and fitness business owners. There are about 25 of us from all over the world who meet three times a year, and we use a Google group to chat between meetings. Every couple of months we each write down our successes and share them with each other. It really helps to share successes with people who can relate to what you're doing and understand and celebrate those successes with you. I love that part of having a positive community, no matter what its mission.

Brainstorm solutions. When you're at a fitness plateau, or you're not getting support from your husband or family for the changes you want to make, or you just need some fresh ideas for what to cook for dinner, it's great to be able to talk to other people who are doing similar things. They may have been through it before. Even if they haven't, they can help you think of possible solutions to your problem.

My Challenge to You

My challenge to you is to share your story, invite others to join you on your fitness journey, and create your own supportive community. Having read this book, you now have more knowledge than most of the population when it comes to the truth about getting healthy and fit. I challenge you to help others and to spread the good word. In fact, I believe that if you've had success with my program and your life has been changed, you have an obligation to teach what you've learned and empower others to change their lives. Even if you're just starting out on your journey, sharing your knowledge and your motivation can transform those around you.

> **"** *Even when you have those frustrating moments, other people have that too, and there's a community you can look to and talk to, and they'll get you past it."*
> — Tina

The first part of the challenge is to share your story with as many people as you can. Don't underestimate the effect your story can have on other people. You might do it through a blog, an email, a Facebook post, a phone call, or a face-to-face conversation—whatever you feel is the best way to communicate your message to your audience. Just share from your heart and say, "This is what I've done, and this is how it's benefited me." As part of that, you can invite people to join you on the journey. You can also invite people to join you when they ask you what you've done to get the results you have, why you're so excited about your workout program, or why you just ordered what you did at the restaurant. When people notice what you're doing and ask about it, they are often looking for answers that will help them make a change. You can respond by inviting them to join you for a workout or lending them this book.

However it works out, you'll begin to teach them all that you've learned and begin to mentor them in their fitness journey. Through teaching others, you'll increase your own understanding and grow your own knowledge as well.

The other part of the challenge is to find at least one partner. I'd recommend you do this as you're starting my program, so that you have the benefits of that support for your own transformation. It could also be something that happens once you share your story and other people see your results. This could be a highly motivated person, or it could be someone you're going to mentor. You can't convince someone that they need to change, but once they've made that decision, you can help them along. If you're interested in organizing a bigger group and starting a *Fit Moms for Life* community, that's even better! Visit *fitmomsforlife.com* to find out how to get involved.

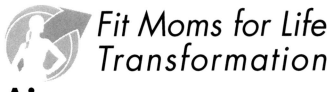

Fit Moms for Life Transformation

Aimee

Despite hating cardio—and hating me the first day she came to MamaTone—Aimee is one of my most consistent clients now, and she always keeps me laughing.

Aimee's story: "I only gained 18 pounds when I was pregnant with my daughter, because I was really sick the whole time—like, vomiting all day, every day. And I lost all of that within the first two weeks after she was born. But then I thought it was my license to finally be able to eat. I was nursing, and I thought I could have all these extra calories. And you don't go out of the house a lot and you're in your nice comfy clothes.... I didn't really notice the weight coming on. But it did. I weighed more when I met Dustin than I did the day before I gave birth.

"I decided I would Pilates my way back into shape going two or three times a week. I liked it, but it wasn't getting me to where I wanted to be. I decided to try MamaTone. I went to class and I hated it. At the end I told Dustin, 'I hate you, I hate this class, I hate everybody in here, and I'm probably never coming back.' And then I threw up.

"But I could see that even though it was hard, it was a structure that I could do. I also liked that Dustin really knows his stuff. He talks about something, like burst training, and the next week there's an article in *The New York Times* about how effective it is."

Aimee's nutrition tips: "I hate saying this, because Dustin was on my case for months—but keeping a food journal really helps. You have to be realistic about what you're actually eating. Also, uncooked cookie dough counts. Eating fries off your kid's plate counts. Samples count. I was making the rounds at Costco and Whole Foods thinking it was okay to eat half a cookie because it was a sample. Then I would wonder why I wasn't losing any weight."

Aimee's advice to you: "Weigh yourself every day. I know there are people who say only do it once a week. But daily weigh-ins let me understand and expect fluctuations in my weight."

Read more of Aimee's story at *fitmomsforlife.com/aimee*.

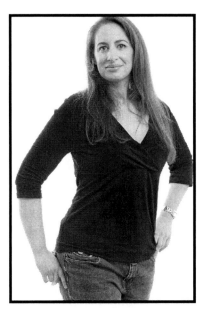

Aimee, 38, mother of one. 5'6", 160 pounds. Aimee has made a real turnaround in her attitude toward exercise, dropping 47 pounds in the past year.

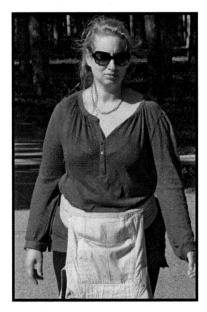

Fit Moms for Life Communities
North Dakota

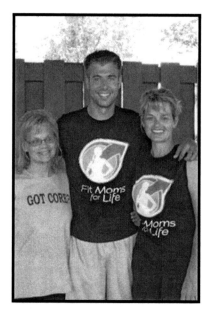

Fit Moms for Life communities are thriving in North Dakota. Patty and Kim both subscribe to the *Fit Moms for Life* DVDs. They've each organized groups of women to get together for workouts based on the DVDs.

Kim runs one group called Casselton Fit Moms for Life, and another at her church called St. Peter's Fit Ladies. Membership of the two groups overlaps, with five to nine girls and women ages 9 to 63 coming to each meeting. Each group meets once a week to do a *FMFL* workout. Kim adds in additional workouts from the *Buns, Guns, Back & Shoulders* DVD, wall-sit challenges, and 500-rep workout challenges sometimes to keep it interesting. They also held a "Biggest Loser" contest within the group.

Me with Kim and Patty from North Dakota, two leaders of Fit Moms for Life communities.

Patty leads a group of five women in Page, N.D., who work out together at 6 a.m. every weekday morning in their school's weight room. Another 40 women are part of Patty's *FMFL* Facebook group—they don't live close enough to join the workouts, but they share recipes, workout tips, and encouragement. Patty's group does strength training Monday, Wednesday, and Friday, and cardio and core on Tuesday and Thursday. Patty also does 500-rep challenge days, which are a group favorite.

Kim and Patty both said accountability is one of the biggest benefits of the *FMFL* community. Patty said, "I have heard many, many times that if I wasn't going to meet the group, they would not be working out; and because I know they're counting on me to be there to lead them in the workout, I have to be there—so it works both ways." Kim also told me that the members of her groups support and encourage each other. They are gaining strength and knowledge and improving their health.

Your Transformation

Remember Kristin, the mom on the airplane at the beginning of this book? We witnessed her realization that she needed to take better care of herself so that she could be at her best for her family. Perhaps you've had a similar moment of clarity while reading this book. Let's take a look at what Kristin did after that "aha!" moment, and what her life looks like a year later.

Kristin made it through that stressful day of travel alone with three kids. She and her husband got a night out in Florida as she'd been hoping, and over dinner she told her husband some of what she'd been thinking about on the plane. She told him that she didn't know exactly what she needed to do, but that something had to change and she was going to need his support. He agreed that she had seemed stressed out and unhappy lately. He hadn't realized how much of a burden she was carrying. They agreed that once they got home, they would start to make some changes.

She heard about the *Fit Moms for Life* DVDs from another mom at her kids' school. She signed up, bought a stability ball and some dumbbells, and started working out at home a few days a week while her toddler napped in the afternoon. It felt good to be able to lift those heavy weights. She often surprised herself when she was able to do the exercises that had looked so daunting the first time she'd seen the mom on the DVD do them! She hadn't thought she had time to work out, but she could put a load of laundry in the washing machine, do her workout, move the laundry to the dryer, hop in the shower, and be done before her son woke up. Her husband took over some chores she'd always done, so that she could take that time for herself in the afternoon. Maybe she was spending less time online and watching TV, but she didn't really miss it.

Through the *Fit Moms for Life* DVDs, Kristin was also learning more about nutrition. She started to change how she ate and how she fed her family. By planning meals in advance and cooking things in larger quantities, she was able to avoid last-minute fast-food dinners and give her family higher-quality food every day. All that planning also meant fewer trips to the grocery store, which was a big time-saver.

As Kristin got stronger and took better care of herself, she gained self-confidence and spoke up for herself more. She worked up the nerve to talk to her siblings about their parents and their increasing need for assistance. They all agreed to chip in to pay for some help. That took a weight off her shoulders. She still stopped in to see her parents a couple of times a week, and they all enjoyed their time together much more than when Kristin was so stressed out.

Some of the other moms in the neighborhood noticed that Kristin was losing weight and looking happier, so they asked her what she was doing. She let them in on her secret. Several of them decided to get together for their workouts twice a week. Their kids played while the moms worked out. (They took turns being on "kid duty.") They got in the habit of emailing each other almost every day, sharing recipes and tips, achievements and frustrations. When Kristin hit a weight-loss plateau, her friends helped her stay motivated and keep up her hard work. They brainstormed changes she could make, and eventually she got back on track.

Getting ready for their annual spring trip to Florida this year, Kristin pulled some cute summer clothes out of the attic. These were clothes she hadn't worn since before her first baby! She's down 25 pounds and is changing the shape of her body, and feeling stronger than she ever has. Her husband is certainly enjoying the results, too. Not only is Kristin looking great, but she's happier, more confident, and more positive about life. He can't keep his hands off her.

Kristin's transformation started that day on the airplane. When will you start yours? What is it going to take for you to start to turn your life around and get into the best shape of your life?

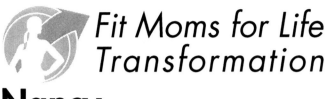

Fit Moms for Life Transformation

Nancy

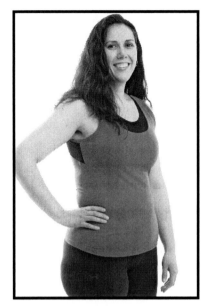

Nancy pulled out all the stops to turn her life and her health around and has made an amazing transformation.

Nancy's story: "My biggest issue has been a problem with body image. I used food as a way to help me feel better about myself. I was anorexic in middle school. I had been bullied about my weight, and I thought, 'I'm just going to take control of my life.' I stopped eating, and I exercised nonstop. I got through that, but I hadn't really figured it out.

"Once I had kids, I really let myself go, as they say. I thought I was being a great mom by doing everything for my kids, but I was running myself ragged. I was 240 pounds and disgusted with myself. About two years ago, I hit bottom. My father passed away after several years of steady decline in his physical ability and health. He was in and out of the hospital. I saw that in my future, and that was completely unacceptable.

"I decided to hit this from every direction. I looked at the food I was eating, how much water I was drinking, and how much sleep I was getting. I started building my support team, because I knew I was going to have some really dark roads to go down. I have a strong relationship with God, and I needed that higher power to get me through it. I joined Overeaters Anonymous, which is a 12-step program that helped me get a handle on my emotional eating. And I started doing Dustin's exercise program.

"I'm really a different person now. I told my husband that people treat me differently. He said, 'No, actually, you're treating other people differently.' He's completely right. I never used to make eye contact, and now I do. My posture is much better. I used to cave in, try to hide. It has been a really nice transformation. I'm happy where I'm at now."

Nancy's advice to you: "You need to realize that you have value. You can change your life right now. It doesn't have to be like this. It's up to you, but if you can do little tiny baby steps along the way, you could be an ecstatic person two years from now."

Read more of Nancy's story at *fitmomsforlife.com/nancy.*

*Nancy, 39, mother of two.
5'8", 170 pounds.
Nancy lost 70 pounds and
overcame her emotional eating
to find happiness.*

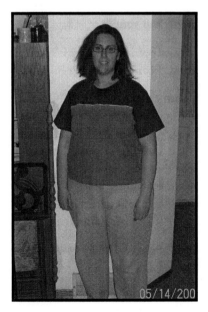

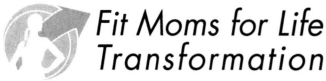

Fit Moms for Life Transformation

Tiffany

Tiffany lost the weight from her first pregnancy and some extra weight she had been carrying to get into the best shape of her life, before getting pregnant with her second child.

Tiffany's story: "I gained about 50 pounds in my first pregnancy and had only lost about 10 of them. My friend had lost weight through Dustin's boot camps, and she has four kids, so I figured if she could make time to do it and get results, so could I. I was working full time as a nurse, so I would either go to boot camp or do a *Fit Moms for Life* DVD at home before work. I lost about 10 pounds a month and after about five months, I was in the best shape I've ever been in, besides maybe when I was in sports in high school. Once I was doing it, feeling good about myself, and seeing results, it wasn't really hard. I looked forward to getting up early and working out and eating well throughout the day.

"Everyone wants to know what you're doing. I work in a big hospital, so I see lots of different people, and every day someone would comment and ask me what I was doing. Sometimes people don't like to hear that I'm doing it just by eating right and exercising, because it seems too simple.

"Shortly after I got to my lowest weight, I got pregnant with my second child. I can't wait to get back to working out at Fit Fun Boot Camps!"

Tiffany's exercise tips: "One: Use heavy weights. Women think they're going to bulk up and get big, but I definitely got very small lifting really heavy weights. And building muscle helps burn more calories. Two: Burst training is great. I'm not a long-distance-anything person, so I love that you can burn so many calories doing something for just a few minutes. Three: Work out with others. That group support is huge. I feel like it held me accountable to show up, and that people were going to see if I wasn't doing the work and wasn't eating right."

Read more of Tiffany's story at *fitmomsforlife.com/tiffany.*

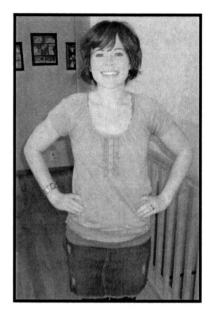

Tiffany, 30, mother of two. 5'4", 139 pounds. Tiffany lost 51 pounds and took nine inches off her waist following my program.

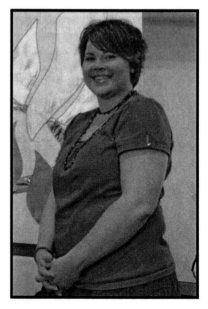

APPENDICES

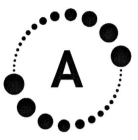

Fitness for New Moms and Moms-to-Be

If you're pregnant, thinking about getting pregnant soon, or recently had a baby, this discussion is for you. (If that's not you, perhaps you know someone who could use this information.) I really encourage you to make a plan for how you will exercise as your pregnancy progresses and once you have your baby. Staying healthy during pregnancy is going to set you up to get back in shape and feel like yourself again more quickly after the baby is born.

I've probably worked with around 50 moms through their pregnancies—including some who were already working out with me when they got pregnant, and others who started early in their pregnancies—and none of them have had any problems continuing the exercise program. The moms who already had older kids have all told me that the pregnancy when they stuck with my program was their best one. During their pregnancies, they say they're feeling better and have more energy, and they don't gain as much weight. Afterward, they get back into shape more quickly.

My recommendations are based on what I've read and what I've seen work for women with healthy pregnancies. However, I'm not a doctor and I don't know your specific situation. Please check with your doctor about whether there are any risks to your specific pregnancy that would mean you need to be more cautious.

Myths About Fitness During Pregnancy

There are a lot of myths and misconceptions about what women should do in terms of diet and fitness while they're pregnant:

"You can't exercise when you're pregnant." There was a time when medical professionals believed that women basically had to lie in bed all day from the time they found out they were pregnant. That was probably because there was so little understanding of what was going on in the woman's body and with the developing fetus, and of course there was a lot of fear about doing anything that might jeopardize the baby. Now we know that it's perfectly safe for women to stay active during pregnancy—with some precautions as I'm going to list below. Exercising while you're pregnant will benefit your health, limit your weight gain, and increase blood flow throughout your body. You can do both strength training and cardiovascular exercise without worrying that it will be bad for your baby.

"You can't lie on your stomach or back when you're pregnant." This is one of many misconceptions about specific things you can't do while you're pregnant. It's true that as you get further into pregnancy, there are risks associated with lying on your back for a prolonged period—basically, the weight of your uterus can put too much pressure on a major vein that carries blood from your legs to your heart. But lying on your back for a few minutes to do an exercise is very unlikely to have any negative effect. Lying on your belly becomes uncomfortable at some point during the second trimester, but it doesn't actually carry any risks for you or your baby. I'd recommend just seeing how things feel. When something starts to feel uncomfortable, find alternate exercises you can do to work the same muscles.

"You're eating for two!" Some women think that being pregnant gives them free rein to eat whatever they want, whenever they want—because they're now eating for two, right? But if you look at how much your developing baby actually needs in extra calories each day, it's really more like you're eating for about 1.2 people. So you're eating about a fifth more than you normally would, or about 300 to 400 extra calories a day. You can increase your portion sizes a bit, or maybe add an extra small meal a day. If you're eating the right foods, your hunger level should be a pretty good gauge.

"The weight will just fall off after the baby is born." This is a myth that survives because it ends up being true for some lucky women. It's certainly not the norm, and you can't count on it happening—even if it's happened for you before. There are a lot of different things that come into play. Hormonal differences from one pregnancy to the next, your age, whether you breastfeed, how active you were in pregnancy—those are just some of the factors. The bottom line is that you should expect to work hard to lose the weight. Don't put on extra weight thinking it will be easy to lose once the baby is born.

Fitness Considerations During and Before Pregnancy
Before conception. When you're trying to decide whether it's the right time to get pregnant, I think the most important question fitness-wise is whether you're comfortable with your current weight and feel that you are in control of your body. This is especially true for women who already have one or more children, and maybe haven't gotten back to their pre-baby weight or at least to a weight where they feel comfortable. I've had a lot of clients come to me after their second or third pregnancies.

They hadn't lost the weight from their first baby before they got pregnant again, and they really struggle with that compound weight gain that's landed them 50 or more pounds over where they were before their first baby. Of course, many doctors will tell you not to start trying to conceive if you're more than 50 pounds overweight, because that extra weight can make it harder to conceive and can also introduce risks during your pregnancy and childbirth. So for fitness and health reasons, my advice is to wait until you're at a healthy weight that is comfortable for you.

During pregnancy. There is definitely a changing understanding these days about what you can and should do while pregnant. The advice you'll get from doctors today is very different from what your mother was told when she had you, which was probably to stop engaging in any vigorous activity. If you had an exercise and fitness routine before you got pregnant, there is really no reason you can't continue doing it. If you were fairly sedentary before you got pregnant, this probably isn't the time to start something intense, but I would encourage you to start walking or doing some less intense strength training. It will still be better than nothing and will help you keep your weight gain under control. Check with your doctor and listen to your body. If it feels like it needs to rest, give it that rest. Pregnancy is not the time to see how tough you are and to push through your discomfort. (Save that for labor!)

When one of my clients gets pregnant, I'm usually one of the first people to know. In the first trimester, there really isn't that much of a difference. The biggest thing is morning sickness and nausea. Some women feel pretty fatigued in their first trimester, which can make it hard to stick to the exercise routine, but the pregnancy doesn't affect what they can do in their workouts. The second trimester is when things start to change a little bit. As I mentioned above, this is when it may get uncomfortable to lie on your stomach and you may have to start altering some exercises. As you get into the third trimester, obviously your belly's getting a lot bigger, and it will start to get in the way of some exercises. Some women feel short of breath or, again, get fatigued easily toward the end of their pregnancy.

You may want to cut back on high-impact exercise and bouncing if you're feeling less stability in your joints, but I've seen moms continue to work out pretty intensely into months eight and nine. You may want to drop it off just a little bit, depending on how you're feeling.

Precautions About Exercising During Pregnancy
First of all, talk to your doctor. Let your doctor know what your exercise patterns are and ask if there are any changes you should make or things you should look out for while you're exercising. (If your doctor is anti-exercise in general and tells you not to exercise at all while you're pregnant, you might want to find out whether he or she is up to date on the research.)

One thing you should know is that your body produces an increased amount of a hormone called relaxin during pregnancy and afterward. It can stay elevated for up to 12 months after pregnancy, depending on how long you breastfeed. Relaxin makes your ligaments, joints, and tendons a lot looser, which is important for childbirth, but it can also make you susceptible to injury while exercising. You might need to be careful with intense exercise that requires lateral movement, jumping forward, stopping, and other exercises that create a lot of momentum. I haven't had any moms have issues with it and get injured, but it is something to be aware of so that you don't push yourself past what feels comfortable with that type of exercise.

Another important precaution in pregnancy is to avoid overheating. You shouldn't be working out during the hottest part of the day or in a lot of humidity. Wear cool clothes, work out in the morning, and be sure your body temperature doesn't get too high. Stay hydrated! You also want to avoid any exercise where you have to hold your breath—that can create an oxygen debt that's not safe for you or your baby.

I already mentioned this, but I'm going to say it again because it's so important: **listen to your body.** If something doesn't feel right, don't do it. If you're just working hard and your muscles are sore, that's totally fine. Definitely take a break if you're feeling light-headed, dizzy, shaky, or like you're overheating. The people I actually get most concerned with are the athletes who are used to pushing their bodies to the absolute max. It's tough to get them to back down in intensity when they're pregnant.

Finally, you should never try to lose weight while pregnant. I see this with a lot of women, especially if they haven't lost the weight from their first baby. This is not the time to lose weight or go to a low-calorie diet. You have to accept that you're going to put on some weight for a very good cause. Be thankful for the baby that's growing inside of you and do your best to eat as healthy as possible. The healthier you are in pregnancy, the easier it will be to get back in shape after the baby is born. So don't look at this as a time to lose weight.

Post-Partum Fitness: Getting Your Pre-Baby Body Back

How quickly you can start to exercise again after giving birth will depend on a lot of different factors. You always want to check with your doctor. But generally, if you didn't have a C-section, you can exercise as early as three to four weeks after childbirth. If you had a C-section, you need more time to recover, so it'll probably be more like seven to eight weeks. You can start walking and maybe doing some body-weight exercises even within the first week, if you feel okay. But by eight weeks, most women can be back to intense exercise. Of course, how quickly you can bounce back to high-intensity exercise also depends on how fit you were to start with and how much you exercised during your pregnancy.

For the first couple of months, your main focus should be getting your core strength back. Your abdominal area has been through a lot, and for some women it comes back better than others. You have to work on the deep core muscles first. They've been stretched and weakened. So you want to hit those front planks, side planks, and vacuum exercises pretty hard to start. Up until five or six months post-partum, I would avoid crunches altogether. (See the box on page 170 about abdominal separation.) Work on those drawing-in exercises, rather than crunches or leg lift motions, because those are only going to make things worse if your deep core muscles aren't ready for them.

Every new mom wants to know how long it's going to take to get her pre-baby body back. Again, it really depends on a lot of things—two big ones being whether you maintained your workouts during pregnancy and how much weight you gained. I can promise you it will go more quickly if you've been working out for your whole pregnancy. If you were on bed rest or just not exercising while you were pregnant, it's going to take longer. What I've seen is anywhere between two months and eight months for most moms to lose the weight

> *Having an infant who napped and nursed, it was hard finding when I could fit the workout in. To be honest, I ended up tweaking my son's schedule so I could make it to class on time. That's how important it was for me to get there."*
>
> – Jody

when they get back to my programs. Some might take as long as a year to get back into the "skinny jeans." Your weight loss might also depend on how quickly or slowly your hormones go back to normal levels, which can be related to how long you breastfeed. Breastfeeding keeps some hormones at elevated levels, like relaxin, as I already mentioned. I know my mom always said that breastfeeding took the weight off her after each of her pregnancies, but some women actually won't lose the fat until they stop breastfeeding. Everyone is different. Don't get discouraged if your weight isn't coming off as quickly as you want. Stick with the program. Continue eating healthy. Stay active. Try to get enough sleep—as hard as it is those first couple months. Stress and lack of sleep are two of the biggest contributors to weight gain. So try to get some naps in if you're up all through the night with the baby. And minimize stress the best you can. Accept any help offered by your family and friends if it will help you to get some rest and reduce your stress level.

The other piece of the puzzle for new moms trying to get back into shape is just figuring out how to fit exercise into the routine while you're taking care of a baby. Especially with your first child, it feels like a lot to juggle, and it can be hard to plan anything around an infant's schedule. Honestly, you have to decide you're going to do it and make it happen. Maybe you can start working out at home when the baby is sleeping, or incorporating your baby into your workouts at home, like in my *BabyTone* DVD. Try bringing the baby with you to the gym—I can't tell you how many newborns have slept through my programs in their car seats at the edge of the room. As your baby gets older, you might be able to use gym childcare services or trade childcare time with another mom who wants a little time for herself, or—once you're sleeping through the night—get up before anyone else in the house to get in your workout. There is always a way to make it work if you make it a priority.

Abdominal Separation

Many women experience abdominal separation (diastasis recti) during pregnancy, and need to be especially careful about strengthening their deep core muscles post-partum. You can check for abdominal separation by doing the "finger test." Lie on your back with your knees up and your feet on the ground. Put one hand behind your head to support your neck as you crunch up just far enough to get your shoulder blades off the ground. At the same time, use your other hand to feel the middle of your abdomen where the rectus abdominis muscles split apart. As you crunch up, you're probably going to feel a gap in between the abs vertically. It's normal to have somewhat of a gap there, especially right after pregnancy. But if the gap is more than two fingers wide, that's a problem. In the long term, we want to see a gap of one finger's width or less. I've worked with women who had gaps up to four fingers wide. Strengthening your deep core muscles is the most effective way to bring those muscles back together, and doing crunches and other outer-ab work will only make it worse. Depending on how severe it is, some women need surgery to repair that, but with good attention to deep core strength you may be able to heal the separation yourself. If your gap is more than two fingers wide, talk to your doctor about the options available.

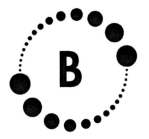

Documenting Your Journey

10-Year Plan Exercise (described on pages 16-18)

Write out your negative vision of your life 10 years from now if you continue with your negative habits:

Write out your positive vision of your life 10 years from now if you make this transformation:

Positive Affirmations (described on page 20)

Write five to 10 positive affirmations below:

Goals (described on pages 28-30)

Write your goals for fitness and other areas of your life. Check that each goal is written in a way that is specific, measurable, attainable, and reasonable. For each goal, indicate the time frame (for example, daily) or deadline (for example, March 1).

Goal	S	M	A	R	Time Frame/ Deadline

Body Measurements (see instructions on page 38)

Date						
Weight						
% Body Fat						
Chest						
Waist						
Abdomen						
Hips						
Thigh						
Arm						

Fitness Tests (see instructions on pages 40-42)

Date							
Front plank (seconds)							
Push-Ups (reps)							
Burpees (reps in 90 seconds)							
Wall sit (seconds) Note any weights held							
Cardio endurance (mile run/walk time)							

3 Day Food Journal

Date:	Date:	Date:
Breakfast	Breakfast	Breakfast
Snack	Snack	Snack
Lunch	Lunch	Lunch
Snack	Snack	Snack
Dinner	Dinner	Dinner
Snack	Snack	Snack
Water	Water	Water

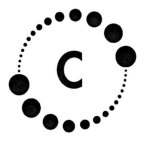

Resources for More Information

Mindset
Positive thinking: Works by Tony Robbins. See *tonyrobbins.com*.

Nutrition
Food journal/calorie-counting websites:

- *livestrong.com*
- *calorieking.com*
- *loseit.com*
- *sparkpeople.com*

The Complete Book of Food Counts by Corinne T. Netzer (8th edition, Dell, 2008)

Food Rules: An Eater's Manual by Michael Pollan (Penguin, 2009)

A Consumer's Dictionary of Food Additives, 7th Edition: Descriptions in Plain English of More Than 12,000 Ingredients Both Harmful and Desirable Found in Foods by Ruth Winter, M.S. (Three Rivers Press, 2009)

Tracie Hittman Fountain's website: *itsyourplate.com*

Wilderness Family mayonnaise: *wildernessfamilynaturals.com*

Nutrient Timing: The Future of Sports Nutrition by John Ivy and Robert Portman (Basic Health, 2004)

Eat This, Not That Restaurant Survival Guide by David Zinczenko and Matt Goulding (Rodale Books, 2009)

Food, Inc., 2008 documentary directed by Robert Kenner

Truth About Six Pack Abs by Michael D. Geary: *truthaboutabs.com*

Cheat Your Way Thin by Joel Marion: *cheatyourwaythin.com*

Isabel De Los Rios' website: *thedietsolutionprogram.com*

Strength Training

The New Rules of Lifting for Women: Lift Like a Man, Look Like a Goddess by Lou Schuler, Cassandra Forsythe, and Alwyn Cosgrove (Avery Trade, 2008)

The Female Body Breakthrough: The Revolutionary Strength-Training Plan for Losing Fat and Getting the Body You Want by Rachel Cosgrove (Rodale Books, 2009)

Raising Healthy Kids

Child of Mine: Feeding with Love and Good Sense by Ellyn Satter (Bull Publishing, 2000)

ellynsatter.com: Division of Responsibility in Feeding section

Two Angry Moms *(angrymoms.org)*, started by two moms upset about school lunches. They made an award-winning documentary that is available for groups to use to host their own showings.

Youth Strength Training by Avery Faigenbaum and Wayne Westcott (Human Kinetics, 2009)

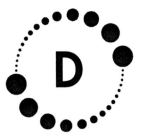

Frequently Asked Questions

Mindset
What if I don't believe in myself?

Just start telling yourself that you will succeed, even if you don't believe it right away. Positive self-talk is crucial if you don't believe you can do something. Tell yourself that all the times in the past when you failed were just practice runs for today, when you will begin the journey toward success. Say it out loud! Find others who will support you and believe that you will succeed, and stay away from people who criticize and belittle what you are trying to do.

One powerful technique is to start your own blog and post pictures and updates from your journey. You can get a free blog at *wordpress.com.*

How do I stay motivated?

Celebrating small successes is huge, especially at the beginning of a new program. If your goal is to lose 100 pounds and after six weeks you have lost five, celebrate those five pounds instead of looking toward the 95 you still have to get rid of. Find ways to celebrate that don't involve food. Reward yourself with a massage, a new pair of workout shorts, a pair of shoes, or a good book.

What is the biggest key to lasting change?

Having the big picture in mind is necessary when you go from starting a program to making it a lifestyle. If you have a big enough "why" in your life, the "how" becomes a lot easier. Remember, the people you surround yourself with will play a crucial role in lasting success. If you make initial changes but keep yourself in the same environment as before, that environment will likely bring you right back to where you started.

Nutrition

How many calories should I be eating to lose weight?

There's no one right answer to this question—it's trial and error. The range I see for women is somewhere between 1,400 and 1,900 calories per day. The surefire way is to do your food journal very thoroughly for one week and figure out how many calories you're consuming. Assuming you were maintaining your weight with that consumption, I would recommend dropping it by 300 to 400 calories per day. I wouldn't drop more than 500 calories suddenly, because that's a big change for your body. First see how your body responds to 300 to 400. If you aren't losing weight after a month, then maybe cut another 100 calories out per day.

Try not to go below 1,400 calories, or maybe 1,300 if you're a smaller woman. That's getting to the point at which your body's barely getting the energy that it needs, and it's going to start to conserve energy and store fat. You don't want that to happen. If you're blessed with a good metabolism and have a really active lifestyle, you may be able to maintain your body weight at 2,500 calories. That can work, but for weight loss, you should try for about a 300-calorie deficit.

Do you recommend eating egg whites or whole eggs?

I used to believe that egg whites were the only thing you should be eating, but with the research that's been coming out on cholesterol and fats, I've changed my opinion. By eating just the whites of the egg, you significantly cut back on the cholesterol, fat, and overall calories. But we actually need good fats in our diets, as we discussed in Chapter 5, and egg yolks provide those. It turns out that most of the nutrients are in the egg yolk, too. (With grass-fed, free-range, local eggs like I encourage you to buy, the yolk is even more nutrient-rich.) If you want to increase your protein intake without adding fat, you can add egg whites, like making an omelet with two full eggs and two additional egg whites. But don't shy away from full eggs altogether.

Can I still drink coffee?

Coffee is one of those things people really hate to give up. I don't drink coffee myself, because I don't like to have anything in my life that's addictive (meaning that I would suffer an adverse reaction if I didn't have it). So I'm a little bit biased against drinking coffee, but if you drink it in moderation, it's not going to do you any harm. Caffeine is the most-used drug in our culture. It's actually been shown to improve exercise performance, and might even bump up your metabolism a little bit when you have it in moderation. Of course, the problem is that most people don't have it in moderation. One, maybe two cups of coffee in the morning or one during the afternoon, assuming you don't put too much sugar and milk in it, is fine. (Look out for coffee creamer, which is laden with chemicals and sugar.) So enjoy your coffee, but don't drink pots of it. You could also switch to green tea and get a smaller dose of caffeine and some great antioxidant and metabolism boosting effects.

What do you think about frozen microwave dinners?

I think they're okay once in a while, but the problem is that most people who use them have them way too often. One good thing about them is that the meal is portioned out for you. Generally they're going to be between 300 and 400 calories, which is about the right amount for a small meal. Unfortunately, they're high in sodium because they're so processed. And they have an ingredient list that's eight lines long in really, really small print, which is never a good sign. A lot of them are also high in fat. If you're going to get a frozen microwave meal, try to get a higher-protein one, with lower carbs and an average amount of fats in it, and use it as backup when you don't have a better option. If you need it in a crunch, it's probably better than fast food, but it's not something you want to do on a regular basis. If you're in the habit of eating a lot of microwave dinners, I'd suggest you try to make your own. Prepare several servings of a meal like chicken, broccoli, and maybe some brown rice or sweet potato on Sunday. Store individual servings in reusable containers in the refrigerator or freezer, so that you can heat it up the same way you would a store-bought meal—except in this case, you'll know what's in it and it will be much better for you.

What do you think about protein bars?

Pretty much everything I said about store-bought frozen meals applies to commercial protein bars as well. They can be good as a backup, but most of them contain a lot more carbohydrates than I would like to see and not as much protein as you should get in a meal. Many of the lower-calorie protein bars contain fake sugars, which I don't recommend you consume. There are some healthier bars out there that just contain dried fruit and nuts. If you are a big fan of protein bars, try making some of your own—you can find recipes online that are based on protein powder and use natural sweeteners.

Eating healthy can be so expensive. Do you have any suggestions?

There are a lot of different ways to save money on your groceries. One is planning ahead so that you know what you need and buying things on sale or in bulk. You can buy local products in bulk from a farmer and split the food with friends or family members. That's an especially good idea for meat products and a lot more cost-effective than buying grass-fed meat in the grocery store. I recommend buying fresh fruits and vegetables when they are in season and the prices are lower. For things that are out of season, frozen vegetables or fruits will usually be cheaper than fresh and are just as nutritious. Of course, cutting out coupons and watching the prices at different stores are other ways to save some money. But you have to keep that to a level where you're still being efficient with your time and gas, and not, for example, driving all the way across town to save 50 cents on milk. In Chapter 5, I mentioned organic foods and shared the Dirty Dozen list, which is a good place to start if you want to reduce your exposure to toxins but can't afford to buy everything organic. Finally, the other big way to save money on food is to use what you buy and not waste food. The typical American family spends close to $600 a year on food that goes rotten.[1] By planning ahead, buying just enough, and eating what you have before you buy more, you should save a lot.

I feel like I'm doing everything right, and it just isn't working. What can I do?

I'd say I get this question from maybe 10 percent of my clients at some point. For at least half of them, the truth is that they aren't following the program closely enough to get the results they want. Usually, they're not eating as well as they should be. But the other 5 percent, the ones who really are following the program and aren't getting results, are the ones who keep me up at night.

I don't have all the answers to this, but there are a few things that might be going on. I'd recommend getting your hormones checked, ideally by a naturopath or another doctor who will work with you to figure out how to fix any problems. Some people do need medication, but I think most of those hormonal imbalances can be fixed through proper eating if you have the right guidance. See Tracie Hittman Fountain's website, *itsyourplate.com*, for more information.

Another thing that can keep you from getting results is an undiscovered food intolerance or allergy. A lot of people have intolerances to different sorts of foods that they aren't aware of, because their reactions are not severe and may not show up on an allergy test. Gluten is an issue for a lot of people, as is dairy. Peanuts and tree nuts can cause people problems. It can be really hard to figure out what it is, but the best thing to do is to eliminate the suspected food for a three- to four-week period and really monitor your body to see how you're feeling. If it feels like you're digesting food better or if your weight-loss results improve, you may have identified an intolerance. Then reintroduce it and see if things go back to how they were, just to be sure that the food item you removed was the culprit.

It could also be stress. High levels of stress increase your cortisol levels. Cortisol can increase your body fat. Lack of sleep goes right along with that. If you're not getting enough sleep, that can cause problems.

Toxicity is another issue that can interfere with weight loss. I don't pretend to fully understand toxicity, but certain toxins in your body can inhibit the release of fat into your bloodstream. You can try going to a diet that is less processed and more organic, but it's pretty much impossible to escape all the toxins in our modern life.

Clearly, there are a lot of things that could be at play when people who need to lose weight can't, even though they're doing everything right. It's a frustrating process, but you've just got to keep your head up and keep trying different things. I would like to believe that most people in this situation can ultimately discover and solve their problem. Keep in mind that even if the weight isn't coming off like you want it to, you're improving your health in other ways by following my program and making healthier choices.

---

1 Jones, Timothy W. "Food Loss and the American Household." redOrbit.com April 4, 2006.

Exercise
Can I work out every day?

I would recommend giving your body one to two days of rest between intense workouts. Rest can be defined differently by different people. I like to call it active rest. So if you're going to go for a leisurely bike ride with your kids, I would consider that a rest day. Maybe you go for a walk, or take a gentle yoga class, or move around a little bit in the swimming pool. But you really need to give your body a break from strength training and high-intensity or high-impact activities like jumping and burst training. If you really want to exercise every day, you can also alternate upper-body and lower-body strength training workouts so that the muscle groups get a day off even if your whole body doesn't. As I described in Chapter 9, if you're doing that, I recommend you pair those workouts with alternating core and burst training sessions so that you don't do either of those every day, either.

I see a lot of people get really gung ho about exercising because they feel so good doing it. Your body can get away with it for a while, but you're going to start to burn out mentally, and eventually it will take its toll on your body, too. You start to plateau, you get injured more, and you don't really increase your strength levels as much. You also get tired more quickly. Sometimes if you're in a rut and you're doing a lot of exercise, the best thing to do is take one week off completely and get kind of reenergized, physically and mentally. Then get going again, but give yourself some time to recover between workouts.

I just can't find the time to work out. How do I fit it in?

Time is one of the few things that is distributed evenly in this world. No matter who you are, you only get 24 hours every day and you have to use them to the best of your ability. If you're thinking, "I don't have enough time," I challenge you to make a chart and track how you use your time for a few days. Account for every minute or at least every 10-minute chunk of time, and figure out what you're doing throughout the day. Chances are you're probably spending at least an hour watching TV, surfing the web, playing games on Facebook, or something like that. That's not very productive—and I bet it's not even that relaxing in terms of relieving stress or getting the endorphins flowing, like exercise would.

It comes down to making your health and fitness a priority. I talk a lot about putting yourself first and believing you're worth it. Once you believe that, you're going to find the time. You may have to get creative. I know single moms who have their kids the whole time—for them, finding time for themselves can be very tough. But it is possible if you make it a priority just like eating, brushing your teeth, seeing your friends, and whatever else you make time for. Do it.

A lot of people find they become more efficient with their time when they start exercising. They have more energy and less grogginess throughout the day, so they're more productive. Even though they're taking those 30 minutes to an hour for themselves, they get a lot more out of the day.

I'm lifting heavy weights and I feel like I'm bulking up! Help!

There are a couple of things that could be going on here. A lot of times our minds play tricks on us. As you get stronger and start to feel muscles you didn't feel before, you might start to think the muscles are getting bigger when they're actually just getting harder. I have clients who swear that they're getting bigger, so I remeasure them and they're always actually a little bit smaller than their before measurements. I think it's just a psychological thing for a lot of people.

But if you feel like your clothes are getting tighter or you've done measurements and you really are getting bigger, the problem may be that you're developing some muscle but not getting rid of body fat. For most people, this indicates a nutrition issue more than an exercise one. Focus on eating the right quality of foods at the right time in the right portion sizes, and you should start to see the body fat melt away and your stronger, smaller muscles appear.

How can I motivate my husband or significant other to exercise?

I wish I had a great answer for this question, because it would help a lot of people and would probably make me a lot of money. The best thing I can tell you is to just set the example and hope he will decide to follow. You can't change another person, so just focus on changing yourself.

I've seen hundreds of these situations, because I've trained so many women. Many times their husbands really become impressed when their wives don't just lose weight, but start to get stronger and fitter and gain confidence in themselves. A man who has watched his wife try other diets and exercise programs before might be understandably skeptical of the "latest and greatest" fitness kick. Then it becomes clear that this program is different; his wife is making lifestyle changes and sticking with them. Sometimes the husband was used to being the fit one and decides he has to try what his wife is doing. Sometimes the husband is out of shape and may start to think he has to change too, to keep up with her. I think he's intimidated, especially if his wife has lost a lot of weight, and that's what motivates him to get started. A good percentage of husbands will start asking what you're doing or showing signs of interest at that point.

But you can't pressure him. You can only explain what you're doing and why you're doing it, and then live it. I hope he will eventually follow you and join you, but I can't guarantee it.

Can I still go for long runs?

If you're the type of person who just loves to run or do another form of steady-state cardio, I'm not going to tell you to stop doing that. I know a lot of people who really love that kind of exercise and get a high from it. I don't want to tell you not to exercise if that's something you enjoy doing. Just be sure to incorporate strength training and burst training into your routine, because that steady-state cardio is not raising your metabolism or strengthening your muscles significantly. You're also going to find that strength training, core training, and burst training will all improve your running and increase your speed. One or two days of a longer run is fine as long as you're getting those other components in.

Is it bad to work out when I'm still sore from the last time?

My rule of thumb is that as long as you don't have sharp pain and it's been a couple of days since the workout that made you sore, working out is just fine and will probably help with the soreness. If you have sharp pain of some sort, that's not good and you need to rest. But if it's more of a dull ache or tenderness of the muscles, you should be fine working out again. Listen to your body as you get warmed up and start the workout. Most people report that they feel a lot better after that second workout loosens the muscles up.

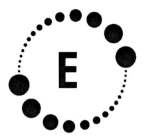

Dustin's Workout DVD Programs

Fit Moms For Life
www.fitmomsforlifedvds.com

Made just for moms, this series of 12 DVDs will help you stay fit and fabulous. The DVD begins with a five-minute warm-up, then moves on to a 30-minute fat-torching and muscle-toning strength workout. After that, you'll do eight minutes of burst-training cardio, then a 15 minutes tummy-toning workout. Add five minutes of stretch time and then, of course, feel amazing! Each DVD features a special healthy cooking segment and interview with Dustin, as well. With each DVD, the workout gets a little more challenging, helping to keep you motivated and moving

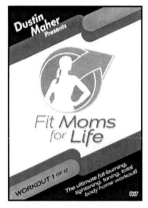

BabyTone
www.babytonedvds.com

Short on time? Of course you are—you're a new mom! With this DVD set, no need to take time away from your little one to fit your exercise time in. These workouts incorporate Baby so that getting-in-shape time can also be bonding time. Brilliant!

Includes two DVDs
- One: Interview, warm-up, two total body baby carrier workouts, baby weight lower body blast workout, tummy tightening baby workout
- Two: Warm-up, two baby weight total body toning workouts, fat dropping burst cardio workout, stroller workout demonstration

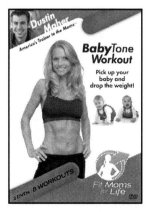

Buns Guns Back and Shoulders

www.bunsgunsworkoutdvds.com

Target your trouble spots with this set of DVDs packed full of workouts that focus on toning up your buns, thighs, arms, and back. With each workout lasting only 8-16 minutes, it's easy to fit one into your super-busy schedule every day.

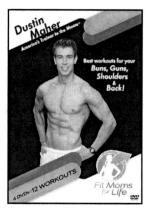

Includes four DVDs

- One: Thighs and buns - four workouts to target your lower half
- Two: Guns - four workouts that specifically tone the arms
- Three: Shoulders and back - four workouts to shape the shoulders and tighten the back
- Four: Interviews with the four women featured in the workouts

Ultimate Buddy Bootcamp

www.buddybootcampdvds.com

Getting fit is better with a buddy! With four fat-burning, muscle-toning workouts meant to be done with another person, you'll never be short on motivation. Get laughing, get sweating, and get fit!

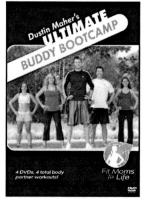

Includes four DVDs

- One: Interview, warm-up, strength training, cardio, core, stretching
- Two: Warm-up, strength training, cardio, core, stretching
- Three: Interview, warm-up, strength training, cardio, core, stretching
- Four: Warm-up, strength training, cardio, core, stretching

Got Core

www.gotcoredvds.com

Target your core with this set of DVDs packed full of workouts that focus on toning your abdomen. Tone your stomach, strengthen your back, improve your posture, and decrease your back injuries with this DVD and a stability ball.

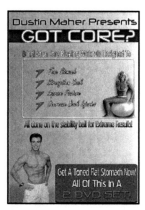

Includes two DVDs

- One: Interview, warm-up, and core workouts level one to four
- Two: Warm-up and core workouts level five to eight

About the Author

Dustin Maher has been a personal trainer since 2004. The first program he created, MamaTone Fitness, is a fat loss program for stay-at-home moms in the Madison, WI, area. As moms started to get results, demand swelled for a similar program for working moms. Dustin created the early-morning Fit Fun Boot Camps, which soon spread to 11 different locations serving women and men of all ages.

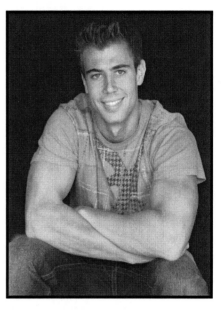

Requests began to flood in from moms around America and the world wanting the eating and exercise programs that Dustin was putting together to achieve such amazing results. This spurred the birth of the *Fit Moms for Life* monthly work out DVD program. Thousands of women from around the world work out to the DVDs which feature average everyday moms who have achieved amazing results through Dustin's program. These DVDs allow Dustin to train any mom, anywhere, anytime.

Since then Dustin has created many more DVD programs all designed to get ultimate fat loss and body transformation from the comfort of your home.

With the success of the DVDs, small groups of women began to form in communities around the world to do the workouts together, building lasting friendships and accountability.

Dustin's mission is to help one million moms get plugged into local *Fit Moms for Life* communities by the end of 2015. If you would like to start your own community, visit *fitmomsforlife.com* to learn how.

Dustin is the oldest of four kids and has a very close relationship with his mom, which is why he feels so passionately about helping moms. After growing up in Elk River, MN, Dustin earned a bachelor's degree in Kinesiology (Exercise Science) at the University of Wisconsin-Madison.

Dustin has appeared on nearly 100 TV shows, can be heard regularly on public radio, and has appeared in numerous newspapers and magazines. He travels extensively giving speeches and workshops to groups of all sizes while still training hundreds of clients in the Madison, WI, area.

Besides working long hours, Dustin enjoys many activities including: lifting weights, biking, hiking, frisbee golf, Scrabble, ping pong, traveling, spending time with friends, watching reality TV, attending seminars, and reading at least one non-fiction book per week.

If you are looking for a keynote speaker or someone to do a workshop on topics related to motivation, exercise, nutrition, or behavior change, you can email Dustin at *dustinmaherfitness@gmail.com*

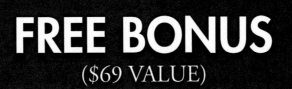
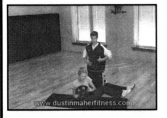
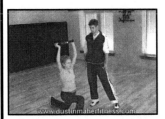
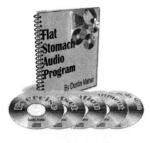
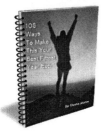

BUY A SHARE OF THE FUTURE IN YOUR COMMUNITY

These certificates make great holiday, graduation and birthday gifts that can be personalized with the recipient's name. The cost of one S.H.A.R.E. or one square foot is $54.17. The personalized certificate is suitable for framing and will state the number of shares purchased and the amount of each share, as well as the recipient's name. The home that you participate in "building" will last for many years and will continue to grow in value.

Here is a sample SHARE certificate:

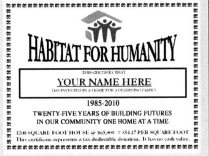

YES, I WOULD LIKE TO HELP!

I support the work that Habitat for Humanity does and I want to be part of the excitement! As a donor, I will receive periodic updates on your construction activities but, more importantly, I know my gift will help a family in our community realize the dream of homeownership. **I would like to SHARE in your efforts against substandard housing in my community!** *(Please print below)*

PLEASE SEND ME _____ SHARES at $54.17 EACH = $ $_____

In Honor Of: _____

Occasion: (Circle One)   HOLIDAY   BIRTHDAY   ANNIVERSARY

   OTHER: _____

Address of Recipient: _____

Gift From: _____   *Donor Address:* _____

Donor Email: _____

I AM ENCLOSING A CHECK FOR $ $_____ PAYABLE TO HABITAT FOR HUMANITY OR PLEASE CHARGE MY VISA OR MASTERCARD *(CIRCLE ONE)*

Card Number _____   Expiration Date: _____

Name as it appears on Credit Card _____   Charge Amount $ _____

Signature _____

Billing Address _____

Telephone # Day _____   Eve _____

PLEASE NOTE: Your contribution is tax-deductible to the fullest extent allowed by law.
Habitat for Humanity • P.O. Box 1443 • Newport News, VA 23601 • 757-596-5553
www.HelpHabitatforHumanity.org

CPSIA information can be obtained at www.ICGtesting.com
Printed in the USA
LVOW052103171111

255461LV00004B/8/P